The
BABY-
MAKING
BIBLE

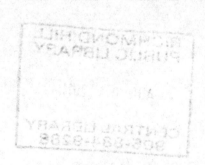

The BABY-MAKING BIBLE

Simple steps to enhance
your fertility and improve your
chances of getting pregnant

Emma Cannon

with Charlotte Edwardes

This edition first published 2010 by Rodale
an imprint of Pan Macmillan, a division of Macmillan Publishers Limited
Pan Macmillan, 20 New Wharf Road, London N1 9RR
Basingstoke and Oxford
Associated companies throughout the world
www.panmacmillan.com

ISBN 978–1–9057–4456–5

Copyright © 2010 Emma Cannon

The right of Emma Cannon to be identified as the author of this work has been asserted in accordance with the Copyright, Design and Patents Act of 1988.

3 5 7 9 8 6 4

A CIP catalogue record for this book is available from the British Library.

Book design by Emma Ashby
Illustrations by Juliet Percival *www.julietpercival.com*

Printed and bound in Great Britain by CPI Mackays, Chatham ME5 8TD

This book is intended as a reference volume only, not as a medical manual. The information given here is designed to help you make informed decisions about your health. It is not intended as a substitute for any treatment that you may have been prescribed by your doctor. If you suspect you have a medical problem, we urge you to seek competent medical help.

Mention of specific companies, organizations or authorities in this book does not imply endorsement of the publisher, nor does mention of specific companies, organizations or authorities in the book imply that they endorse the book.

Addresses, websites and telephone numbers given in this book were correct at the time of going to press.

Visit *www.panmacmillan.com* to read more about all our books and to buy them. You will also find features, author interviews and news of any author events, and you can sign up for e-newsletters so that you're always first to hear about our new releases.

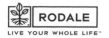

We inspire and enable people to improve their lives and the world around them

*For my parents, whose great love
conceived five daughters.*

And for my grandmother.

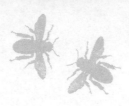

Contents

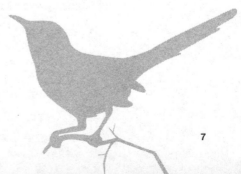

Foreword by Dr Tim Evans

For those of us who come from an evidence-based Western science background, Chinese medicine can seem bizarre. 'But how *exactly* does acupuncture work?' my medical colleagues will ask. I always reply honestly: 'I really don't know. I just know that, in many cases, it does.'

My own conversion to the benefits of Chinese medicine was based on proof. For twenty years I had suffered from hay fever. While my friends enjoyed the arrival of summer, I would be behind closed doors and windows, my nose streaming, my eyes red and inflamed, and my mind befuddled from the antihistamine drugs.

Seeing my extreme discomfort, an acquaintance suggested acupuncture. This was ten years ago and acupuncture, as a treatment, was still very much on the periphery. I agreed to give it a go. This was not so much due to open-mindedness, but more out of desperation.

I tried not to be too judgmental as the needles were carefully placed at various sites on my body. It is difficult to accept that such a simple procedure can achieve miraculous results after you have spent a large chunk of your education studying conventional medicine. After a couple of treatments, however, the symptoms were certainly less debilitating. After four treatments I was 'cured'. Now, every spring I return for a top-up session and, as such, have not required nasal sprays, eye drops or sedating medication ever since.

With that cure came my conversion – at least to the possibility that there was an unexplored world out there of treatments and cures that we still knew very little about in the West. When I set up my own private general practice, I took this knowledge and introduced it to my patients. I worked alongside acupuncturists, osteopaths, reflexologists, nutritionists, hypnotherapists and massage therapists. I was determined to embrace all aspects of health care in what is now commonly termed 'an integrated approach' to medicine.

I think we were ahead of the curve in adopting this change in attitude. A general 'softening' towards complementary and alternative medicine (CAM) became established. Acupuncture was tested in high-quality clinical trials and the results sent waves through the medical community. In the area of fertility in particular, Chinese medicine showed itself to be an incredible force. Where Western methods were sometimes failing, Chinese methods were getting results.

In Western medicine we are constantly challenging, updating and enhancing our understanding of disease and, as a result, modifying its treatment. Similarly, we must always consider the benefits that other forms of medicine might offer. Happily, this integrated approach is now more readily accepted by the medical profession as a whole.

It is this integrated approach that Emma Cannon adopts with her patients and has now made available in *The Baby-Making Bible*. This book is not just enormously practical and helpful, offering readers advice to help them on their fertility journey, but it is written with warmth, experience and a profound understanding of the power of both Chinese and Western medicine.

My hope is that in years to come I will be updating this foreword, to include more and more areas where acupuncture and the theories of Chinese medicine have been proven by Western medical trials to be effective. Meanwhile, in partnership with courageous practitioners like Emma Cannon, I will continue to provide my patients with the best care that both Western and Eastern medicine can offer.

Dr Tim Evans, September 2009

Introduction

'Expect a miracle'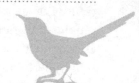

You may have picked up this book because you are just starting to think about having a baby, or you may have been drawn to it because you've been longing for a baby and want to know what you can do to improve your chances of conceiving. Whatever the reason, one thing that it's important for me to say at the outset is that I cannot help you actually make a baby – that part is down to you. What I *can* do, however, is share with you the secrets of my success with the many patients I have treated for fertility over the years.

People come to me for different reasons. Some want to ensure the healthiest possible 'fertile ground' in which to grow a baby naturally; others, who are about to embark on IVF treatment for the first time, want to do the best they can to improve their chances, while those who are on their second or third attempt at IVF are looking for help to make it work. And some come simply with unexplained infertility.

Part of my motivation for writing this book came from my desire to give my patients and my readers advice on what they can do to enhance their fertility. Indeed, the question I am most frequently asked by my patients is 'What can I do to help myself?'. My heart always sinks when patients tell me how they have asked this question before and have been told that there is little or nothing they can do to increase their chances of conceiving. My view is that there is always *something* you can do to help yourself and that the very act of taking matters into your own hands means that couples often feel more assertive and more positive. Of course, not everything can be fixed by *doing* and sometimes it is a case of just *being*, but this too can be done in a guided and useful way. I am not talking about false hope here, I believe that we can have hope when we discover that we *do* have options and that there *are* positive steps we can take throughout the fertility journey.

Whether you are trying to conceive naturally or you are undergoing fertility treatment, the period of time before you conceive gives you a key window of opportunity in which to evaluate where you could make small changes to your diet, activity levels and general lifestyle to optimize your fertility, create a more perfect environment in which to grow a baby and increase your chances of a healthy pregnancy.

The power of an integrated approach rooted in Chinese medicine

My background is in acupuncture and my area of expertise is in treating infertility and gynaecological conditions, and I am privileged to work alongside some of the UK's leading medical specialists in these areas.

Acupuncture forms part of Chinese medicine, the oldest continuously recorded treatment system for human illness and ailments. For a practice that dates back more than two thousand years it is surprisingly sophisticated and the insights and wisdom this ancient style of medicine offers are both complex and significant. Chinese medicine uses a range of treatments including acupuncture, herbalism, tinctures, dietary advice, massage and exercise such as tai chi and qigong, in order to maintain health as much as to treat disease.

There is overwhelming evidence that Chinese medicine can play a significant role in treating infertility, gynaecological problems and balancing hormones, and it is these principles that I draw on in my work with my patients in my London practice. But I do not work in a 'bubble'; rather Chinese medicine forms the framework for the baby-making plan I offer patients, with Western diagnosis and results forming a crucial part of my knowledge and understanding of how I can help someone improve their health. I work closely with my Western medical counterparts in the field of gynaecology and infertility to support their treatment. This mix of influences, along with a desire to keep techniques up-to-date and modern, means that my practice sits very much between the two worlds of Western and Chinese medicine, drawing from each of them for the greater good.

My experience of working with practitioners such as gynaecologist and obstetrician Jeannie Yoon has been particularly thrilling. I believe the way we work together is a true example of integrating medicine for the good of the patient. Generally speaking, couples experiencing fertility issues don't necessarily want to be put straight on to medication, and so most are delighted when someone like Jeannie encourages them to try an alternative approach before heading down the intervention route. When medication is necessary then patients are of course offered it, but when other complementary methods could be tried first, then patients want reassurance from their medical practitioner regarding the therapies and complementary practitioners involved in their care, which Jeannie offers. Patients also want to know there is dialogue between practitioners.

One occasion particularly springs to mind, when a delighted mother turned up with her teenage daughter who had been suffering from an irregular menstrual cycle. The mother was impressed that Jeannie had suggested she saw me first rather than be put straight on the Pill, as is often the case. Within three months of my treating her, she had a regular bleed. Together we have countless cases such as these and in my experience this is the kind of medicine that people tell me they really want.

So, while personally I am devoted to endorsing natural methods to enhance reproductive health, I take a wide perspective and my aim always is to offer the best treatment available. I have developed and refined my approach over the past fifteen years, and while its roots are firmly in Chinese medicine, my method has been heavily influenced by my work with practitioners of Western medicine too. It cannot be denied that medical advances – such as IVF – have been astonishing in recent years. But no matter how exciting scientific leaps can be, we must still remember that some problems can be resolved in the simplest of ways. Some doctors are quick to reach for the fertility medicine, yet not everyone who has problems conceiving needs IVF, and this is, I believe, where my approach is crucial.

My view is that it is essential to spend time (and I do realize that in some cases there is little time) getting as healthy as possible in both body and mind as part of the process of conceiving. I want to give you the opportunity to gain a 360-degree insight into your health which can reveal simple obstacles that may be overlooked when someone is automatically fast-tracked to IVF. I have seen this happen in my own fertility clinic in London: patients decide to overhaul their health before IVF, and then conceive spontaneously.

My approach to fertility

My integrated approach to health and fertility is always with one aim in mind, and that is to optimize a patient's overall health and wellbeing in order to enhance their fertility and maximize their chances of getting pregnant. And this is what I will offer you in this book – a personalized baby-making plan that you can follow, safe in the knowledge that it works – it has worked for countless patients in my clinic (I have a very high pregnancy success rate among patients) and it can work for you too. I believe in an integrated approach to healthcare and in empowering couples to make adjustments to their life that may help their condition, give them confidence and encourage them to understand that they have an important role to play in preparing for conception.

The main aim of Chinese medicine is to create balance and harmony in the body, and this shall be my starting point in this book. I always start the same way with my patients, and that is how I will start with you here: by slowing down, taking the time to ask some key questions and by applying my custom-made 360-degree approach to your life and your health (see pages 85–107).

Rather than simply treating superficial symptoms, I will encourage you to look at the 'whole you', and demonstrate how you can take your wellbeing into your own hands and start to address any underlying health issues you may have to eliminate disharmony and create wellness. Often lifestyle issues, medical issues, emotional distress or trauma can lead to illness and blockages which threaten the balance and throw the system into disarray. We will examine these issues, and also look at the importance of the menstrual cycle, and examine any gynaecological disorders you may have, the role your hormones play, your diet, your lifestyle, your sex life and your emotions with the aim of creating harmony in all these areas, to make sure the 'engine' is working, that the 'fuel' is good and that your mind is on board. As you experience a deeper connection with your body and all that it is capable of, I hope you will gain a sense of pride about being in the best possible health to conceive a child and a desire to be as healthy as possible – in both body and mind.

I will take you by the hand and lead you through my baby-making plan – a plan that encompasses every aspect of your life – with the aim of showing you that the changes you make are worth the effort and that, with time, you can become healthier, stronger and ready to conceive a baby. Much of the information I offer has been handed down from generation to generation, woman to woman, mother to daughter, practitioner to practitioner, healer to healer. Chinese medicine is still used, alongside Western practices, in hospitals in China today. The information I am going to share with you has stood the test of time. Some of my tips may sound strange or old-fashioned, or perhaps too simple to be effective, or even too much like hard work. I urge you to make the effort and to understand that sometimes it is the simplest changes that can have the biggest impact on our health and fertility.

My four-month baby-making plan can help you:

- understand your body better and discover what 'fertility type' you are; this gives you the knowledge you need to help get your body in balance and ready for conception
- balance your hormones and achieve optimum health and wellbeing
- improve the quality of your cervical mucus (essential for successful fertilization)
- improve and thicken the endometrium (lining of the uterus) to prepare for an embryo to implant
- manage gynaecological conditions such as PMS, amenorrhoea (lack of periods), ovulation problems, endometriosis, PCOS and embryo implantation issues

- prepare for IVF and learn what you yourself can do to help support you through the procedure
- promote egg quality, prepare for egg transfer and aid fertilization and implantation in IVF
- learn to manage and overcome stress through other complementary therapies, such as yoga, meridian tapping, practising affirmations and visualization.

It can help your partner:
- improve sperm quality – count, motility and morphology
- improve his overall health
- become more involved and connected with the baby-making process.

My own route to Chinese medicine

In addition to an undergraduate degree in acupuncture, I followed the traditional training in Chinese medicine, studying under several true masters. They taught me the importance of clinical intuition and expertise which complemented the technical and theoretical practice I was gaining at university in London. I decided to specialize in women's health, fertility and children very early on.

In my first acupuncture job I worked with John Tindall, a physiotherapist and acupuncturist who knows how to push boundaries safely to help patients learn the spiritual lessons that are sometimes necessary in the healing process.[1] I also met Nanette Greenblatt, an 'intuitive', who had an enormous impact on my work. She advised me to work with both Western *and* Eastern medicine in order to help keep complementary methods alive and to ensure they were always up to date. This became the fundamental principle in my integrated approach. I look for ways to build good working relationships with GPs and specialists, and to find common ground.

In 1999, I was introduced to Dr Tim Evans, a general practitioner who would later become the royal physician. He shared my vision for integrated healthcare in which Western and complementary medicine are practised side by side. He was about to launch a new clinic and asked me to join his team.

Tim Evans has an all-inclusive, integrated approach to health and for this clinic he envisaged a practice where patients would not necessarily be put straight on medication, but rather all treatments, complementary included, would be considered. All the while, patients could remain safe in the knowledge that science was not being overlooked. He created a clinic full of specialists who were open-minded and ambitious – not for themselves, but for the benefit of their patients.

In 2004, together with highly respected consultant obstetrician Michael Dooley I founded the Fertility Support Clinic at Westover House. Our aim was to provide an integrated approach, caring for and managing gynaecology, fertility and pregnancy patients. Michael treated me as an equal – something that can be unusual with doctors; he knew I wasn't trying to *do* his job, but to support it. He gave me the confidence to approach Western medicine practitioners and to demonstrate to them the benefits of acupuncture and other complementary therapies.

Many of our clients then were following a path that is so typical of the approach to conceiving a baby today. Some had little time for sex or were saving intimacy for the 'fertile' time of the month. In some cases, conception was taking a long time to happen, but the conditions were a long way from what Chinese medicine would hold as 'healthy' and 'fertile' ground.

In Chinese medicine, the health of both the male and the

female at the time of conception determines the health of the child. An 'irregular' life – eating erratically, eating while working, rushing, talking about business, travelling – are all seen as being detrimental to health. Similarly, stress affects the liver and can have a knock-on effect on both libido and mood.

I put all of these factors into my consultations, and Michael Dooley and I began to see the results of changing our patients' lives. This new approach was so successful that I earned the nickname Emma 'the baby-maker' Cannon, and our clinic went from strength to strength.

Then, in 2005, fate dealt me my biggest challenge: I was diagnosed with breast cancer. I was thirty-seven years old and, I'd thought, in excellent health. I was married to the man I loved with two beautiful children and a job that I was passionate about. On paper I had zero risk. I'd had my first child at twenty-seven and breastfed her for two years. I had never taken the contraceptive pill. I'd eaten organic before anyone else knew what it was. I hadn't even used chemical deodorants or worn underwired bras!

The first night after diagnosis was harrowing. I lay in bed, imagining another woman bringing up my children. I tortured myself. I did this for two full nights, and then I gave myself a good talking to: I looked in the mirror and said out loud, 'You need sleep; you need rest. If you don't get sleep you will not get better. If you wake up in the night, you are *not* to think like this. If your mind strays into that pattern of thinking, you must empty your head and go back to sleep.'

Gradually, I began to see my diagnosis in a different light. My surgeon told me that the cancer I had was unusual. It was the type that old ladies usually get – low-grade and non-aggressive. I'd had it so long it had begun to behave aggressively, but it had taken eleven years to do so. Could my healthy way of life have improved my chances? Statistically, younger women get the *most* aggressive cancers.

Another reassuring factor was that I already had in my life the people I would most need to get me through this – from my Western oncologist to John Tindall, an acupuncturist and 'healer', and everyone else in between.

It never crossed my mind not to take the treatment I was offered, first in the form of surgery to remove the lump and the affected lymph nodes. But I balanced this by resting and eating nourishing foods. I took remedies and I recovered fast and without problems.

Then came the chemotherapy: six rounds of it from May to October 2005. This also required mental strength. I approached my great friend and colleague Emma Roberts, who practises hypnotherapy and a technique that involves tapping at meridians used in acupuncture in order to open emotional blockages.[2] I told her, 'I have to believe chemotherapy is going to help me. At the moment I'm afraid that it will poison me. I *want* to believe it is the silver elixir of life, and they are putting it into my veins.' So, before every session, Emma hypnotized me to believe just that. To this day, I have no trauma attached to my treatment and I put that down to a combination of the amazing skill of the chemotherapy nurses and the mental state that Emma helped me to achieve.

I don't often mention my chemotherapy to fertility patients – the two worlds rarely collide – but I can draw on the experience when I explain to them the importance of visualizing what can sometimes be unforgiving fertility procedures as something to help them achieve their goals.

Following each dose of chemotherapy, I had acupuncture. This helped to relieve the nausea and strengthen my blood. Michael McIntyre, the president of the National Institute of Medical Herbalists,[3] gave me herbs to keep me strong and to help my blood count recover. This is important: blood needs to recover after every chemotherapy session so that you are strong enough for the next hit. My chemotherapy was never held up – my blood recovered every time. I attribute this to both the protective nature of the herbs and my visualizations. I visualized my blood at the exact level needed. And then I rested and nourished myself. After each dose, I rested for three days solid. I carried on with my life in between.

Next came radiotherapy, possibly the worst part of the treatment. The hot, aggressive energy that came from the radiotherapy felt to me like a fire. I rebalanced my own energies by meditation, cooling herbal medicines and acupuncture. Under hypnosis, I bathed my body in a cooling, healing light to counteract the raging, burning effects of the radiotherapy.

Again, this experience helped me a lot in my work with fertility patients – after all, there is a need to balance sterile, clinical fertility procedures with something natural, earthy and nurturing. It may not be an obvious parallel to 'unexplained infertility', but I know how it feels to be frustrated with your body, and how to turn around a diagnosis with a combination of Western and Eastern medicine and a hefty dose of mental strength.

My experiences have helped me to empathize with patients' emotional pain, as well as the sense of desperate urgency they feel. I understand the journey: the repetition of the treatment, the way it erodes your time and destroys your freedom. I understand how it feels to let go of the desire to control what you *can't* control.

I have learnt, and have taught patients, how to live in the moment – you can't stray off into what might happen next; you have

Note
Throughout the book, when referring to a Chinese medicine term, I give it a capital letter (Qi or Liver, for example). This is because Liver in Chinese medicine has a far wider meaning than that attributed to the word in Western terms. Chinese medicine ascribes not only function, but also emotional features to organs: the Liver, for instance, is associated with the drive for life, vision and is also connected to the eyes. So when you see the capital letter, we are talking Chinese medicine.

to live with where you are, focus on the present and what you can achieve on any given day. I often refer to the book (and film) *Touching The Void*, in which Joe Simpson, a climber who was left for dead in a crevasse on a mountainside, describes how he crawled on his tummy all the way back to camp. Rather than take on the enormity of his situation, he inched forwards in bite-sized pieces, planning to make it just to the rock ahead, then to the next rock and so on, until he finally reached his goal.

How this book can help you

I have set this book out in such a way that you can start with maximizing your chances at spontaneous (natural) conception, before moving on, if necessary, to the more complicated assisted-reproduction procedures. And my checklist – under the recurring headings, 'Is the engine working?', 'Is the fuel good?' and 'Is the mind on board?' (i.e. do you feel fit to drive?) – will help you to work on your whole system.

In Chapters Two and Three, a diagnostic self-assessment helps you to match your symptoms against a 'fertility type' – these are very simplified versions of those used in Chinese medicine. The aim is for you to correct your type's quirks and bring yourself closer to the 'ideal' in order to conceive without problems. Once you have identified your type – or types (most people have symptoms from more than one) – you can follow the baby-making plan in Part II. I have mapped out the whole menstrual cycle with advice for you to follow under the checklist headings (see above). The plan I have drawn up is based on a twenty-eight-day cycle. You can slightly adjust the first fourteen days, repeating or skipping days depending on whether your cycle is longer or shorter, but menstruation occurs fourteen days after ovulation, so everyone can keep to the second half of the cycle in the way I have mapped it out. All you need do is follow the recommendations for your type or types. I strongly believe that you need to repeat the plan for four whole menstrual cycles to ensure that you are in absolute optimum health for conception.

My patients do have excellent results, and that is exactly the reason why I have chosen to commit this simple plan to a book: I want to reach the widest audience I can so that as many couples as possible have the chance to achieve a healthy conception.

At this point women often say to me: but what about my partner? Does he have a role to play? And the answer is: yes, a big one. You partner needs to be fully on board. He will have to make changes too, but it's all for the benefit of creating a fertile seed and soil in which to grow a healthy baby. With this in mind, I have included a box on sperm on page 46 and a cycle specifically for men on page 196. There are, in addition, many other parts of this book that you will want to share. You can also both visit my website, www.emmacannon.co.uk for more information and advice.

My clients are busy people, as are you, so in addition to my baby-making 'Master Plan' – featuring essential advice on understanding your menstrual cycle, sex, lifestyle changes and tailored recommendations for you – I also offer top baby-making tips along the way, comprising those little things you can do every day while you are trying to conceive, whether it's an affirmation to help keep you focused and positive, a herbal tea to try or a yoga pose to practise. I will show, as demonstrated in my case studies, that taking control of your fertility makes a real difference.

The case studies in this book are based on patients who I have treated over the years. Their names have been changed and in some cases details have been adjusted in order to protect their privacy.

There are Q & A sections throughout the book. Questions were put to a panel of experts in the field of fertility. Half are trained in traditional Chinese medicine and half are Western-medicine trained. Each question was put to the panel and the answers were compiled from the combination of their answers.

The final chapter is devoted to those who are already undergoing IVF or other fertility treatments. During my career, I have treated many couples going through IVF and I've learnt first-hand how acupuncture can benefit this process. I've therefore been disappointed to learn from many of these women just how great the focus is on producing large quantities of healthy embryos at the fertility clinics and how little emphasis is placed on the general health and wellbeing of the would-be parents. This is an area where more of the principles of Chinese medicine should be applied, concentrating on the whole person, rather than just one symptom (in this case, problems conceiving).

This 360-degree approach allows you to take some responsibility in your fertility. It is not a 'band aid' solution; it addresses your health as a whole. That means that, whatever the outcome, this process will help you. I would like to promise everyone a baby, but life simply doesn't work like that. I can, however, promise that you will walk away from this process with better health, more self-awareness and the tools to address areas of your life that have held you back for years. You will also greatly improve your chances of having a baby. Your ability to achieve this really is now in your hands.

Emma Cannon BSc Hons Ac, MbBAcC
www.emmacannon.co.uk

Part I

PREPARING TO MAKE A BABY

Chapter One

A new approach to health and fertility

So, you want to make a baby? I'm here to help and am going to be your personal practitioner. I will take you by the hand and walk you, step by-step, through the process of getting into the best possible health for conception. This is the blueprint of the method I use in my clinic – a method which has helped hundreds of women get pregnant. And now I am sharing it with you.

My approach is underpinned by the spirit and principles of Chinese medicine, a great and mighty system of diagnosis and treatment that has been in use for over 2,000 years. Now you are going to use Chinese medicine to improve your over-all health, your fertility and your chances of conceiving and carrying a baby full-term.

The sceptics among you may well be asking, 'Can you *prove* that your results are because of Chinese medicine?' The answer is simple: when you work with something for long enough, and you hear the feedback from patients and see the results, you don't have to prove anything. Put simply, the proof of the method is in the pregnancy.

Some of my patients have been through what I would

genuinely term as 'ordeals' when it comes to fertility treatment. So they really benefit from a more simplified approach, a life with less stress, better food and regular, loving sex. These are the basic ingredients for human happiness, good health and optimal fertility, and I will give you my key pointers to achieving all of this in this chapter.

Embarking on my baby-making plan

First, you need to be positive. You have taken your health into your own hands and are about to embark on an incredible journey. As you read this book, try to keep in mind the image of yourself as pregnant, and recognize that each step that you take on this journey is a fertile exercise that contributes in its own small way to the greater goal of achieving a healthy conception.

Next, you need to arm yourself with information, starting with this chapter where we are going to talk about general health. Understanding what affects your health is very empowering. It helps you to make choices about how you live, eat and view yourself and your life.

I am often asked why it is so important to be in the best possible health *before* conception, and the answer is that not only will you be more likely to conceive, but you will also increase your chances of a healthy pregnancy and be giving your baby good health for their own life. As obstetrician Gowri Motha says: 'I have always been bemused by the fact that as... women, we spend longer planning the nursery for the baby, than our bodies.'[1]

This chapter looks at everything under the enormous banner that Chinese medicine calls 'health', considering what health actually is, and how the way we live impacts on it. I have divided the many contributing factors into three sections:

- **Is the engine working?** This covers the physical and general lifestyle issues and what is in the environment around us. This is also about optimizing the flow of energy or 'Qi' pronounced 'chi' (see box, page 31) in your body. For more on Qi, see Chapter Two.
- **Is the fuel good?** This covers what you put into and use on your body.
- **Is the mind on board?** This is essential reading – the mind can be a totally unexpected barrier in fertility.

Is the engine working?

Everyone can improve their general health and every woman can learn more about herself by connecting to her menstrual cycle. That's why this book is for everyone wanting to conceive, regardless of whether or not they are having difficulties.

Ideally, you should follow the pre-conception plan (see Part Two) for four cycles, time allowing. You can then continue to follow it while you are trying to conceive, and during any medical treatment. My guidelines are based around the idea of achieving optimal health and attaining balance in the body for conception.

Avoiding overwork

Chinese medicine, which is very much of the 'everything in moderation' school, takes a dim view of overwork. However, as it is all about balance, I am also going to cover 'underactivity' here, as neither is good for your overall health.

There are workplaces where it is culturally acceptable, if not encouraged, to be the first to arrive in the morning and the last to leave. Many women travel great distances to work, where they spend long hours at a desk, sitting with bad

CASE STUDY: A SCEPTIC IN HER OWN WORDS

In 2001, I went to an IVF clinic to find out why I had stopped having periods. I had married six months earlier and I wanted children. I felt my case needed to be investigated.

After running endless tests the doctors were unable to find any reason why I was not having periods. They told me that without assisted conception I would be unable to have children.

I embarked on ovulation stimulation first of all, which did not appear to have any effect, then three rounds of IVF. During the first attempt, the hospital was doing a medical trial. They wanted to find out whether women who had acupuncture during the procedure to transfer eggs were more likely to conceive. All the patients that day had acupuncture and I did fall pregnant, but sadly it ended in a miscarriage. During the second IVF attempt, the trial was still ongoing, but patients were being randomly chosen and were not informed if they had been given sham acupuncture during the procedure. The trial was not ongoing during the third round of IVF. The other two treatments were unsuccessful.

After the third attempt failed, one of the doctors suggested that I have a break from IVF and try alternative therapies. I was sceptical, but I was prepared to try anything once if it meant I might conceive. They recommended I see Emma Cannon and, in April 2004,

I met her. I told her I had not had a period all year and she prescribed a course of acupuncture and her baby-making plan to re-establish my menstrual cycle. I had decided not to do IVF again until September and Emma said she didn't want to rule out the possibility that I could still conceive naturally – but I had my doubts.

I saw Emma weekly for the first month, and then every couple of weeks. In one of our meetings, I burst into tears and asked her, 'Where is this all leading?' I felt another year would go by without having a baby. Emma agreed that it was frustrating that I still hadn't had a period, but she said that my health had improved dramatically and that I needed to stick with it and be positive.

Later that week I was convinced I had food poisoning. When I still felt ill five days later I asked my husband if I should take a pregnancy test, just in case. We were both very aware that it could be a case of false hopes, but, to our utter amazement and delight, the test was positive.

I continued to see Emma once a month for the rest of my pregnancy. When I reached my due date, I saw Emma and told her how heavy and fed up I felt, and asked if she thought acupuncture could get things moving. She did. Two days later, on 15 March 2005, Harry was born.

postures in over-air-conditioned offices. They stop off at the gym on the way home and put their exhausted bodies through a workout with the same mental determination that they apply to their jobs. Then they relax in the steam room, further depleting their bodies of essential energy.

These hard workers are the least likely to take holidays and most likely to turn up at work when they are ill. They tend to override their tiredness with stimulants (such as caffeine, sugar, Red Bull and empty calories), and have trouble getting to sleep. A glass of wine with friends may help, but either way, the knock-on effect of a frenetic mind will be felt the next day, the day after and so on.

Among others, I see bankers, lawyers, doctors, journalists, politicians, actresses, analysts and athletes in my clinic. Often, these high achievers get to the top of their field at a high cost to their fertile health. Those in vocational jobs too, find it hard to delineate between work and pleasure.

Think about how much time you spend on work and going to work. The arrival of a baby requires massive adjustments. If you currently start work at 7 a.m. and finish your day at 10 p.m., it's time to start thinking about what needs to give.

I'm not saying you should give up your job or your ambitions, but I am suggesting you think about how you could make space in your life for a baby. Obviously, there are health benefits to loving your job, but you need to create boundaries. I know plenty of mothers who work hard, yet they still protect the time that they have for their children. You need to focus on this delicate balancing act. Make space for a baby now by making time to get healthy for conception.

The most hardworking are often what we call 'Blood Deficient' in Chinese medicine (see page 121). Blood Deficient types need to rest. Overwork depletes energy.

Simple adjustments can make a huge difference. Dropping the evening gym session and walking to work, if possible, in

WHAT IS QI?

Many cultures have belief systems that are similar to Qi (pronounced chi), particularly in the East. It is like the yogic idea of 'prana' (breath). Qi is the flow of an absolute life force, a universal energy. It is everywhere and it keeps us alive. It is what oils every function in the body and it's what acupuncturists tap into when they place needles into points just below the skin's surface.

As Qi can be a hard concept to understand, I am going to try to simplify the idea for the purposes of this book: I want you to think of it as your overall vitality. The Chinese 'cultivate' and 'balance' this vitality. They do this with diet, exercise, such as tai chi and qigong, and with acupuncture.

In Chinese medicine, one person's vitality and energy can be very different from another's, so you shouldn't compare yourself to anyone else (see page 111). The quality of your Qi comes from a combination of two things: what you have inherited from your parents (see the section on 'Jing' further on), added to the vitality that you have acquired in life. The Qi that has been acquired in life is what we are going to concentrate on. This is the bit you can really change for the better. The Chinese say that you cannot replenish what you have inherited, but you can preserve it in life.

How can you cultivate good Qi (or vitality) in life? You can do this through the food you eat, the exercise you take, in the way that you moderate your life and manage stress and how you balance your emotions. You can even do it through the people with whom you choose to surround yourself – in the same way that certain people can sap your energy, so they can deplete your Qi. And, conversely, some people can have a 'great energy'.

Cultivating better, stronger Qi is a Chinese obsession. Gyms, for example, do not have the widespread popularity in China that they enjoy in the West because pumping iron and pounding the streets to burn calories are considered to be Qi-depleting activities (although this is gradually changing, largely because of the influx of Western business and personnel). You are more likely to see people there standing rod-backed like trees in the park, cultivating Qi from their surroundings by practising tai chi.

Similarly, calorie counting is not big in China. Traditionally, the Chinese diet incorporates a huge variety of foods, and food is medicinal as well as essential and enjoyable. Obesity has not been a widespread public health problem there in the past, although the increasing popularity of Western junk food means that it is becoming more of an issue for the next generation.

So, the aim is to cultivate your Qi and to get it in balance so that there are no obstacles in your path to conceiving. And the recommendations I make in the first three chapters will help you to do this.

the morning instead is a great idea. The morning is perfect for exercise, as you are rested and ready to go. What about an early-morning swim? Or yoga stretches? These are far better than forcing your overworked body through a rigorous routine in the evening when it is ready to collapse. Evenings should be sacrosanct: you need to relax, rest and take care of yourself – and, yes, make space for your baby.

Remember that fertility is a receptive act; it's not necessarily about achieving by *doing*. I like to get my patients away from that frustrating approach – the feeling that they are banging their head against a brick wall in the drive to *achieve* something.

It's also important to take your holiday. Holidays can be a fantastic way to gain perspective (the Chinese see perspective as important in fertility). Some of my patients need to soften, by which I mean they need to let go and be less controlled and rigid, so I send them away to find 'fertile activities': painting classes, writing courses, gardening, cooking – anything that is a complete creative distraction. Fertile activities are those you do, not for results, but for the pure indulgence of it. Often, women find that when they do something totally different, something just for *themselves*, they soften. And this can shift perspective enough for them to start approaching the issue of fertility in a whole new way.

Avoiding being underactive and unfulfilled

Recent research shows that vast swathes of the population do nothing at work. They are bored, unchallenged, untested and stuck. It is a soul-destroying existence, but once you are in the rut, it's hard to escape.

Being unfulfilled has an impact on the whole of your psyche and wellbeing and leads one way: to Stagnation. If you recognize this in yourself follow the plans set out for Stagnation (see pages 138–140).

I often see women who are flushed and frustrated, tears welling in their eyes. They tell me they hate their jobs but have 'hung in there', desperate to get pregnant. I totally understand why someone would stay in a job for the maternity benefit. But equally, if you hate your job, there's a lot riding on getting pregnant *now*, and, if you don't, your unhappiness with your situation can increase tenfold, which is counterproductive: put simply, if you are unhappy in your work, your health will start to suffer. You board a train of negativity that goes nowhere. In the long run, you are at risk of severe frustration, a loss of drive and 'situational' depression.

Sometimes women spend years trying to get pregnant and simultaneously not moving on in their lives without realizing that one is impacting the other. What they need is purpose – to give them a renewed drive for life. According to Chinese medicine, if you have no drive, your vision for the future can be clouded. Vision is essential for conception.

It can also be hard to treat someone who has been stuck in a negative rut for a long time, but the fact that you are reading this book means that you have taken the first step to changing your life around. Here are some tips:

- **Write a bold plan:** 'What do I want to achieve in life, love and with work? What is my purpose in life?'
- **Be creative:** what could you do to complement and 'balance' work?
- **Write a 'gratitude diary'**, concentrating on the good things in your life.
- **Get out of the house:** accept invitations; go for walks; visit a museum; meet someone for coffee.
- **Try a new hobby** – is there something you have always wanted to do? How about something 'hands on' like pottery? Or perhaps you could devote some time to a charity?
- **Look for solutions:** banish complaining and try to think

around the problem. For example, if you don't get on with a colleague, think of ways to improve the situation: keep away from him or her as much as possible; avoid confrontation and try to greet every slight with a smile.

- **Take responsibility for your life:** pick yourself up and give yourself a good talking to – affirmations are great for building up your drive (see page 72).

CASE STUDY: MARATHON WOMAN

One of my fertility patients was a marathon runner who was having problems conceiving. Everything she'd been taught in life was associated with working hard to achieve results. When she didn't achieve what she wanted she just worked and trained harder. It was her firm belief that if you work hard you could achieve any goal; she was very much of the 'if at first you don't succeed… ' mentality. While this approach had served her beautifully in her chosen profession, it wasn't working when she wanted to conceive.

I sat down with her and tried to get her to rethink the way she viewed fertility. Rather than looking at the process in the Western linear sense – 'I ovulate on Day 14 and I should be pregnant on Day 28' – I tried to get her to think in terms of preparation and cycles.

She perceived herself to be in 'peak' health, as did her friends and family. This type of physical fitness, however,

wasn't necessarily the best condition for conception. She was hard, wiry and thin, not soft and receptive. She was very disciplined about health and diet in a way that was almost counterproductive – she felt that she needed to be in firm control of everything around her, including the way her body worked. The idea that she couldn't 'achieve' conception was frustrating her and making her work harder. I really had to coach her to let go of the idea that falling pregnant was like running a marathon.

It took a while, but we really turned a corner when she realized that it wasn't a competitive race to conception. It was with great relief that she finally accepted that, 'If it takes me another six months, my body will be even better rested and better nourished'. She needed to let go in order to conceive, which she did – and she enjoyed the process.

She did conceive and she carried to term.

Managing your stress levels

Stress can be felt by anyone in any situation. It's not the pre-serve of the hard-working, as is often suggested; those who are underachieving can also feel stress, as can those who are struggling to find work or be fulfilled. We all feel stress dif-ferently and, as you will often hear me say, it is unhelpful to compare ourselves to others.

In my practice I see women who are wrung out by stress. Some are locked in to the mentality I talked about in the sec-tion on overwork (see page 28), and every inch of their lives is crammed with high-octane activity.

When we become stressed our bodies adopt a 'fight-or-flight' response, which prompts the adrenal glands to se-crete cortisol (the stress hormone) and adrenaline into the bloodstream. This is a survival reflex. It is essential, however, that our bodies are allowed to fall back into a relaxed state after 'fight or flight' so that basic functions such as heart rate, blood pressure and digestion can return to normal.

Problems occur when the body is not able to resume its normal state because we are trying to 'fight' on many fronts. This is often the case with people who are running insanely hectic lives and trying to juggle too much, and it can lead to chronic stress, exhaustion and, in severe cases, a depletion of cortisol and/or a breakdown.

When I see a very stressed patient, the first step of their treatment is, obviously, to get them to relax. Actually, this is great as the results are immediate; often, I can almost see the zigzags coming off them as they walk out of the door. It is always my aim to completely calm them down to the point where they appear to be walking on cotton wool as they leave. It's not uncommon for me to hear women say: 'I've completely forgotten what I was stressing about.'

Teaching yourself to relax is an essential tool for life – and also for parenthood. So, once you have taken the step of recognizing that your stress levels are too high, there are fantastic and simple therapies in this book that you can use at home, including:

- aromatherapy oils in a candlelit bath
- deep-breathing techniques
- yoga
- qigong
- meditation
- self-hypnosis
- meridian tapping (see page 78)

Obviously, the desire to get pregnant and finding it is not happening for you creates a horribly stressful situation. But you need to learn to manage stress before *it* becomes the problem.

Getting enough sleep

The importance of sleep, I'm happy to report, is an area on which both Chinese and Western medicine are very much in agreement. Sleep is so important. It is essential for life – for survival. Most animals need sleep too, even if, like the giraffe, they nap for a matter of minutes at a time.

A lack of sleep can have a detrimental effect on the normal functioning ability of both body and mind. If you don't get enough sleep you can fall ill,[2] as well as have difficulty healing.[3] It will affect your ability to concentrate, to stay calm and composed and to exercise good judgment. It will also impact on your memory and, consequently, your ability to think. You can go without food for longer than you can go without sleep.

Lack of sleep has also been shown to affect hormone secretion, and although this is an understudied and under-researched area, it is certainly known that lack of sleep and changes in time zones due to travel can interfere with your

JING (OR YOUR 'CONSTITUTION')

Another crucial issue is a patient's Jing, or constitution (also sometimes referred to as 'essence'). A fundamental principle of Chinese medicine is that your health is affected by that of your parents. Your Jing is your ancestral health. You can't do anything to change it, but if you look after yourself, you can maintain good health and can certainly pass better Jing down the generations. Your Jing is the blueprint you will hand down to your baby.

This is not an alien concept in Western medicine, of course. That you can have a 'genetic predisposition' to certain diseases, illnesses and even personality traits is now widely accepted. Studies show, for example, that a child whose grandmother smoked while pregnant may have double the risk of developing asthma compared with one whose grandmother didn't – even when their own mother didn't smoke.[4]

Researchers believe that tobacco alters the genes in the reproductive cells of the foetus, causing changes that are then passed on to the next generation.[5]

The way you manage stress is also crucial. According to Marcus Pembrey, a leading specialist in genetics: 'The mother can pass stress hormones, metabolites or immune cells (lymphocytes) to the foetus while it is in utero. [These are] likely to affect the child's health later on.'[6] And a number of studies by Professor Vivette Glover in the Fetal and Neonatal Research Group at Imperial College, London, found that unborn babies exposed to high levels of cortisol, which crosses the placenta, had double the risk of developing attention deficit hyperactivity disorder (ADHD).

However, by living a healthy, balanced existence, the Chinese believe you can maintain the status quo and pass good health on to your children. To gauge the state of the constitution you have inherited, you need to ask:

- Was either of my parents older than thirty-five when I was conceived?
- Did my parents smoke at that time?
- Did they drink alcohol at around the time I was conceived?
- Did they take drugs?
- Did my mother smoke, drink or take drugs during pregnancy?
- Was my mother very stressed or traumatized during pregnancy?
- Was my mother ill during pregnancy?
- Did she have any serious accidents?
- Am I the youngest of many children conceived in quick succession?
- Did my parents suffer from any hereditary illnesses?
- Do I have grey hair prematurely?

Remember: the answers to these questions do not spell disaster; they are merely a means of charting how you need to take care of yourself. It doesn't mean you are going to get ill, but it does mean it is worth staying in good health and preserving your constitution.

menstrual cycle. All of these factors are crucial for women who are trying to conceive.

In Chinese medicine, it is held that lack of sleep, like too much stress and overwork, can deplete the Qi which, in turn, can be a catalyst for other health problems. Many of the patients I see are Qi Deficient, and many are busy, hard-working professionals who lead hectic lives, cramming every conceivable activity into a tight twenty-four-hour day. The classic complaint is that of feeling tired all the time, barely refreshed in the morning and tired after eating. I work on building Qi reserves: when your Qi is strong you are better able to cope with stress and your body functions better. And sleep helps you to cultivate your Qi.

The story is the same from the Western perspective, and although sleep is not fully understood, it is of increasing interest to Western scientists. Dr Neil Stanley, a sleep researcher and senior lecturer at the University of East Anglia, argues that, 'Good sleep is vital for good physical mental and emotional health – but, unfortunately, we seem to live in a society that has forgotten that fact.'[7] Dr Stanley says that sleep is equal to diet and exercise in terms of good health. 'Poor or inadequate sleep can have serious consequences on overall health and wellbeing and has been shown to lead to lower immunity, poor performance and mood changes.' This falls in exactly with what Chinese medicine teaches us.

Any number of simple factors can affect sleep, from drinking caffeinated drinks too late in the day, to keeping our mind in a frenetic state of activity long after it needs to wind down. I also believe in the old-fashioned idea of being 'overtired'

Q&A

I travel for work and I am often flying long haul, can this impact on my fertility?
Yes, unfortunately this can be a problem, not only for the disruption that long distance travel can have on your menstrual cycle but also for the period of time spent away from your partner. Try to avoid unnecessary travel or try to time it for the period before ovulation if you can.

and how this can affect our ability to sleep, in much the same way that it affects a tantrum-prone toddler.

How many hours' sleep do we need?

Western research suggests that the optimum amount of 'good' sleep for adults of all ages is between seven and nine hours a night. Fewer than six hours a night will affect cognitive performance, according to the study, published in 2007.[8] Between six and seven hours is the minimum that will allow the body to experience the four essential stages of sleep – which are known as N1, N2 and N3 (also called Delta, deep sleep or slow-wave sleep) and Rapid Eye Movement (REM).

But when my patients ask how many hours' sleep they need, I always get them to factor in a 'wind-down' period before bedtime. Don't try to tot up how much you can achieve in terms of working, socializing or exercising before you reach the deadline. It's no good trying to sleep after a hard hour-long session in the gym, a three-course meal or a long stretch working at the computer.

If you operate best on, say, eight hours' sleep, try to make sure that the hour before you go to bed is spent doing something truly relaxing – having a bath, reading a book or practising gentle yoga or meditation, for example. Here are some other suggestions for a good night's sleep:

- Don't eat too late at night. Most of us still tend to have our main meal only hours before bed, but this can wreak havoc on our digestive systems and prevent us from sleeping.
- Don't have serious discussions before bed: you may not be able to digest issues and it may prevent you from 'switching off'.
- Don't work too late, especially not just before you go to sleep.
- Go to bed early – it's better to go to sleep before you

feel tired than when you feel 'overtired'. As my mother always said, nothing good ever happens after one in the morning (with the exception of birth), so try to make this an absolute, absolute deadline.

- Try to keep your bedroom as dark as you can, cutting out as much outside light as possible.
- Only drink coffee between 10 and 11 a.m. and keep tea to a minimum. In the evening, stick to herbal drinks – especially chamomile, which is known to be soothing and calming.
- Sleeping pills can prevent the mind from experiencing all the essential stages of sleep and can, therefore, make you feel more tired in the morning – avoid them.
- Alcohol can have a similar effect on the brain to sleeping pills, so limit the amount you drink.
- Reduce activities that are stimulating to brainwaves, such as the computer and even the television, before bedtime.

CASE STUDY: ELECTRIC DREAMS

Don't underestimate the effect of having too much electrical equipment in your bedroom.

I had a patient who couldn't get to sleep at night and when she did go off, it was lightly. She was getting increasingly exhausted and irritable. I asked her about her sleeping environment, and it emerged that she had more electrical equipment in her bedroom than an outlet of Curry's.

In addition to the TV, she used the laptop in bed, charged her mobile next to her head, and around the bed she had a baby monitor, a radio and a CD player. All were either on or on standby at night, with their little red lights shining into the darkness. I was pretty sure that all the electromagnetic activity would interfere with sleep, so I suggested she unplug it all and see what happened.

Perhaps not surprisingly, she was 'cured' immediately. She subsequently banished all electronics (aside from the baby monitor) from her room.

- Don't use a mobile phone or laptop in your bedroom – electrical equipment produces electromagnetic energy which can stimulate your brain when you are trying to sleep (see Case Study).

What is the best position to sleep in?

The position you sleep in can affect the quality of your sleep, according to sleep researchers. Recommended positions include:

- **the foetal position** – on your left-hand side with your back straight and your knees bent
- **the 'star fish'** – flat on your back in a star shape, which is similar to the yoga position 'savasanah'
- **the 'yearner'** – on your side with your arms stretched ahead of you.

I should add that although sleeping on your back is a recommended position for many, it can encourage snoring in some people. Sleeping on your front can cause cricks in the neck, back problems and pins and needles.

Some women find that pillows help to prop them up. For example, if you sleep on your left-hand side with your right leg hitched up, a pillow under the right knee can provide support for your back. A pillow between the knees in the foetal position can help stop them knocking together. These positions are also very good once you are pregnant.

The principles of exercise

Exercise is a wonderful way to channel frustration, a great distraction and it also releases endorphins, which make us feel better about ourselves. In the context of Chinese medicine it has the benefit of moving Qi and blood around the body (so those who discover they are Stagnant – see page 138 – will benefit greatly). Like everything in Chinese medicine, however, it depends on who is doing the exercise and how much, and it is essential to exercise within appropriate limits.

Women who are used to a high level of exercise, like my marathon runner (see page 34), need to maintain a certain level of exercise because their bodies are used to it. Others, who do very little exercise, will need to start their routine gently. It's important to be in good shape before you conceive (see box on obesity, page 56), as if you are not, it can affect your ability to conceive.

I don't like to see people pounding the streets or exercising to the point of profuse sweating, especially if they are trying to conceive. It may make you feel better in the short term because it moves the Qi around your body, but it is also exhausting. So, once again, we come back to balance. Moderate your exercise according to your own vitality. Listen to your body, and don't go beyond your limits. *Never* exercise to the point of exhaustion.

Good exercise for fertility

The following forms of exercise are all helpful when it comes to fertility:

- **Qigong** – this is particularly good for those who need to build or move Qi (see page 132 for more on Qi Stagnation). See page 192 for more on qigong. Do you need a teacher? It has an effect on the mind and the body and can be practised by anybody, of any age or body type. I have recommended some simple qigong exercises throughout the cycles to get you started.
- **Swimming** – a good gentle exercise for general movement (but don't swim while you are menstruating – as it can make you 'Cold' – see page 112).
- **Yoga** – great for everyone. My colleague Uma Dinsmore-Tuli has provided advice on yoga throughout the book.
- **Walking** – this is beneficial not just for exercise, but also

to get those who feel 'stuck' moving again. It's a good distraction and it's an excellent gentle build-up if you are not used to exercising.

- **Tennis** – perfect if you are moderately fit because it helps the mind to focus and allows you to have interaction while you exercise.
- **Pilates** – encourages core strength, stability and is an excellent preparation for pregnancy.
- **Belly dancing** – something a little different, and particularly good if you are Damp, Blood or Qi Stagnant.

Think about your environment

I had a patient who, when purchasing a new home, commissioned an electromagnetic survey of the surrounding area, as well as the normal structural survey, in case it affected her chances of conceiving. My view is that while I do think it's worth trying to bring down the amount of electromagnetic activity in your bedroom, it is, perhaps, ambitious – and unnecessary – to take on an entire area of London!

There is, however, worrying evidence that our increasing use of chemicals is polluting the ecosystem and having an impact on the normal reproductive function of animals. Tests have shown that a group of chemicals called alkylphenol ethoxylates (APEs), which mimic the hormone oestrogen, cause reduced sperm count in wildlife. APEs are commonly used in cleaning products, detergents, hair dyes, aerosols, rubber and plastics that are not easily biodegradable when they are washed down the drain. And it has been found that fish that swam in contaminated water showed signs of feminization, hermaphroditism and lower survival rates. I therefore urge all the couples

Q&A

Can I keep up my normal exercise, which includes running?

Exercise is a healthy part of everyday life when practised in moderation it can really benefit health. However, running is not considered an appropriate exercise in the post-menstrual phase when we are trying to encourage the blood to flow to the uterus to add implantation. If you are used to running and find it helpful then carry on but tone it down by two thirds.

who see me (and particularly the men) to avoid products that contain APEs.

Many of us live in an urban, modern environment and, short of moving into the deepest countryside, there is little that we can do about the wider usage of man-made chemicals in the world around us. However, each of us can do our own little bit to reduce our level of exposure to the chemicals that some researchers believe could seriously harm us.

If you can't cut it all out, find a balance that works for you – such as limiting harsh chemical cleaners in the house, but occasionally using the dry cleaners. Or perhaps you want to continue having your hair dyed, but are prepared to cut out the fake-tan spray. (Incidentally, I know an eminent Harley Street obstetrician who feels so strongly about not using fake-tan sprays that he tells his pregnant patients he would rather they had a glass of wine and a fag!)

More research is still needed into the effects on our fertility and the health of our babies of toxic chemicals in the environment. However, here are some general tips on the sort of chemicals you may want to avoid[9]:

- **Household cleaning products** A large number of potentially unpleasant man-made chemicals lurk within these, but you can get around this by choosing the natural alternatives that are now widely available. You can also knock up some homemade cleaning products: white wine vinegar (or cider vinegar) dissolves dirt, cleans glass and can even be used to clean wooden floors and toilets. Soda crystals are brilliant for scouring – particularly baths and basins. And they are cheap, too!
- **Insecticides and pesticides** These are dangerous to pregnant women and so, equally, should be avoided by those trying to conceive.
- **Dry cleaning** Try to limit the amount of dry cleaning you have done; when you do have clothes dry cleaned take

them out of the plastic and air them afterwards.

- **Cellophane (cling film)** Cellophane contains chemicals that are oestrogenic and potentially damaging to sperm. These chemicals have also been indicated in breast cancer, polycystic ovaries and endometriosis.
- **Soft plastics** These, again, can leak oestrogen-mimicking chemicals. If you are going to buy bottled water, buy glass wherever possible, or, if you do buy something stored in soft plastic, think about switching the contents to glass jars or bottles. Be especially careful about allowing water bottles in the car to heat up, for the same reason.
- **Aluminium** Be careful about using products with aluminium, such as tin foil (and definitely don't cook with it).
- **Microwave** My view is that microwaves are not good when you are trying to conceive. If you *have* to use one, don't buy second-hand (in case it leaks) and don't stand in front of it when it is on. And never microwave food wrapped in plastic (such as ready meals) or on a plate with cling film over it.
- **Beauty products** Choose natural alternatives wherever possible, and go without make-up occasionally.
- **Nail varnish, hair dyes and fake tans**. If you use any of these, or if you regularly lie out in the sun slathered in some sun creams, you are probably exposing yourself to benzophenones, PABAs, cinnamates and salicylates. There are chemical-free or chemically reduced alternatives.
- **Botox injections** Avoid these altogether; botox is not a good thing to have in your system if you are trying to conceive.
- **Anti-perspirant** Buy deodorants rather than anti-perspirants and check to ensure that they don't contain aluminium. We were meant to sweat; it's part of the

THE IMPORTANCE OF HEALTHY SPERM

We are seeing a marked decline in sperm counts from the early 1990s. One study argued that the average sperm count had declined by 29 per cent in 10 years, comparing figures between 1989 and 2002.[10]

Modern life is a significant factor. Damage is caused to sperm by smoking, and researchers are now focusing on the effects of chemicals found in everyday products such as plastic bottles, sun cream, deodorant and paint.

Another area of scrutiny is anti-androgens, also found in products such as plastics, shampoo and soap and known to be absorbed by body fat. Peter Deadman, author of a number of research articles on male infertility, points out that these 'have been shown to correlate with a higher-than-expected number of abnormalities in human genital development, including smaller anogenital distance,[11] smaller scrotum and penis and an increased likelihood of cryptorchidism[12]... (associated with reduced fertility).'[13]

Men who have a high number of abnormal sperm need to ejaculate regularly throughout the month, so that their sperm constantly regenerates and comes from the back of the testicles. They should not ejaculate daily during the woman's non-fertile time, but in the fertile window every day is fine, starting 4 or 5 days before expected ovulation. Men with a low sperm count need to conserve their sperm, ejaculating every other day during her fertileperiod, starting 4 or 5 days before expected ovulation. They should ejaculate less frequently in the non-fertile time.

Dos and don'ts for healthy sperm:

- **Do** take zinc supplements.
- **Do** cut down on or avoid alcohol.
- **Do** talk to your doctor if you take the antidepressant Paroxetine (also known as Seroxat or Paxil) because research suggests that it increases the levels of sperm with damaged DNA.
- **Do** avoid heat such as steam rooms, and cycling for long periods of time.
- **Do** avoid pesticides.
- **Do** avoid unfiltered city tap water (a study showed lower sperm counts and abnormally shaped sperm in men who drank London tap water. Common detergents were thought to be the cause of the reproductive damage).[14]
- **Do** avoid toxic paints, paint strippers and paint-diluting chemicals – a study of painters found they are more likely to father children with defects of the central nervous system.[15]
- **Don't** smoke – smokers have lower sperm counts and more abnormal sperm.
- **Don't** take recreational drugs – they affect sperm count and increase the risk of birth defects.
- **Don't** use your laptop on your lap – keep it away from your testicles.
- **Don't** keep your mobile phone in your trouser pocket, next to your testicles.
- **Don't** try to conceive shortly after an anaesthetic (in tests on animals sperm damage was 50 per cent higher after anaesthetic enflurane).

elimination process. Try acupuncture and herbal medicine if you suffer from embarrassing sweating odours.

- **Talc** This should be avoided, especially on your underwear or vagina, as it can travel up the Fallopian tubes and affect the ovaries.

Is the fuel good?

The principles of how to eat

I am not a food fascist; food is one of life's great pleasures. If you eat and cook fresh food, your diet will be healthier and you will also probably be more likely to lose weight and be healthy than if you eat processed 'low-fat' or 'diet' foods.

Obviously, it is essential to be in good health for conception, but I think there is a misunderstanding over what actually constitutes a 'healthy diet'. My rules, which are based on the principles of Chinese medicine, are as follows:

- Eat well, eat light, live longer.
- Eat foods that are in season.
- Eat slowly – chew your food properly to aid digestion.
- Eat for your type (you will learn about your type over the next couple of chapters, and I have included recipes and recommendations accordingly).
- Don't eat too late at night; you won't be able to digest your food properly or sleep.
- If you can afford organic food, that's great; if not, stick to buying locally grown produce rather than food freighted from abroad – or grow your own!
- Try not to study, watch TV, read a book or discuss work while eating. In Chinese medicine it is the function of the stomach to digest both thought and food. If you do both at the same time, you are taking the energy away from the digestive function.

- Eat a good breakfast, e.g. porridge made with water.
- Chicken soup is restorative and nourishing (see page 50 for my recipe).
- Don't flood your system with gallons of water – drink when you feel thirsty, when you have a dry mouth, a headache or if you feel dizzy when you stand up.

Throughout the book I have made suggestions for each particular fertility type as to what you should keep in your kitchen store cupboard. In addition to the information here, there are literally hundreds of books on diet, so for something more comprehensive check my references on page 360.

Seasonal food

Eating fresh, seasonal food is obviously not a new idea, but it has recently become a very fashionable issue and it seems many celebrity chefs – Hugh Fearnley Whittingstall, Gordon Ramsay, Delia Smith to name a few – now have seasonal cookbooks. Chinese medicine too, holds great store by the

INTENSIVE FARMING

There has been a lot in the media on intensive farming recently, not just because it is destroying land, but also because of the intense use of pesticides, chemical fertilizers, herbicides, fungicides and insecticides, all of which have been indicated in fertility issues in animals.

Where possible, and I realize this can be the more expensive option, eat the freshest and least-tampered-with options you can lay your hands on and choose home-grown (UK) foods.

It also makes sense to eat a free-range chicken rather than a stressed-out one that has lived an appalling life in dreadful conditions. And once roasted, you can put the carcass to work for your chicken stock, of which I will talk almost incessantly (see below).

importance of life's cycles, harmony with nature and balance, and recommends eating foods that are appropriate for the time of year.

Britain is mostly a cold and damp country; it rains a lot and it's not often warm. Consequently, we need a diet that is warming and easy on the digestion: slow-cooked foods are great – such as oven-roasted seasonal vegetables, soups and stews with wholegrains, such as barley and amaranth. A small amount of raw food in the spring and summer can be very helpful – but balance these with soups. Raw foods are probably best avoided in the middle of winter by all but the fieriest Heat types (see pages 126–129).

Fats – good and bad

Don't be taken in by modern, faddy diets. The word 'fats' has become a bad word and most of us now instinctively avoid anything containing them, whether through fear of weight gain, health reasons or fears about the effects of dairy products when they are consumed in vast quantities. However, there are good fats and bad fats.

Good fats
Monounsaturated fats
These lower total cholesterol and can help weight loss. They are found in:
- nuts, including walnuts, almonds, pistachios
- avocados
- olive oil.

Polyunsaturated fats
These also lower total cholesterol and can be found in:
- fish oil, including salmon and other oily fish (these are omega 3 fatty acids)
- sunflower oil

THE BENEFITS OF CHICKEN SOUP

Hanna Kroeger, who in 1958 opened New Age Foods, the first health-food shop in the United States, was an early proponent of the medicinal properties in everyday food. In her book *Ageless Remedies from Mother's Kitchen,* she asks, 'Why is chicken soup superior to all the things we have, even more relaxing than Tylenol [paracetamol]?' And she answers:

It is because chicken soup has a natural ingredient which feeds, repairs and calms the mucous lining in the small intestine. The inner lining is the beginning or ending of the nervous system. It is easily pulled away from the intestine through too many laxatives, too many food additives... and parasites. Chicken soup... heals the nerves, improves digestion, reduces allergies, relaxes and gives strength.

Throughout history and across the world, chicken broth has been recognized for its restorative properties. It is frequently given to those who are ill, and although often associated with Jewish mothers, it has been as prevalent in Persian and Muslim history and culture, as it has in the Jewish tradition.

All of my patients – even the vegetarians (yes, I do try to convert them on this one thing) – are sent home with a chicken soup recipe to suit their type. I give the base recipe for stock here so that you know where to start, but in the section on types (see pages 108–141) I will describe how to adapt your soup according to your type. You'll also find my friend Victoria's recipe for chicken noodle soup below, which is a jazzier version of the basic soup. It is better to make it with uncooked bones if you can.

Chicken Stock (base for chicken soup)

You can make chicken stock with a single uncooked chicken carcass or bones but it will be improved if you add extra legs, wings and giblets (but not the liver). Or you can use a roast chicken carcass.

1. If you are using a leftover roasted carcass, pull off any spare meat and set aside to use when you make the soup. Next, push down on the carcass until you hear the bones crack, then pull it apart and add to a large stock pot. Use the entire carcass, including any juices left in the roasting pan. If you are using an uncooked carcass or bones, simply squash down into your pot.

Now add to the stock pot:

2 large carrots, chopped

2 cloves

2 sticks of celery

2 bay leaves

2 onions, halved with the skin left on

a sprig of thyme

10 peppercorns

You can also add a leek, spring onions or parsley stalks if you have them in the house.

2. Cover the ingredients with fresh water (preferably filtered) and bring *almost* to the boil (but make sure it doesn't boil). Reduce the heat, until the stock is just simmering, and leave uncovered for 1½–2 hours. Check intermittently and skim off any froth that rises to the surface. If using uncooked bones or carcass, you'll need to cook for longer, 3 to 8 hours.

3. When it is cool, strain the stock through a fine sieve and chill in the fridge. If there is a thick layer of fat on the top the next day, scrape it off.

4. When you come to make your soup, briefly bring the stock to the boil and add vegetables, such as carrots and celery. Finally, add the pieces of roast chicken you set aside. Adapt as necessary using any of the suggestions for your type (see pages 108–141).

Victoria's Chicken Noodle Soup

1. If the stock (above) has been cooked for less than six hours, bring it to the boil for about 20 minutes and reduce for richer, more intense flavour in the soup. Otherwise, it is ready to use and needs to be heated to bubbling point. Next, add the following:

a few dashes of nam pla (fish sauce)

a few pieces of thinly sliced fresh ginger

1 thinly sliced red chilli

a slug of (medium dry) sherry

juice of 1 lime

a few greens, such as cabbage or pak choi (optional)

2. Now cook the noodles (if your noodles are not separated into individual servings, use 3–5oz per person if they are dried, and 4–5oz if they are fresh) in boiling water until they are al dente and drain (or rinse, if preferred). Add them to the soup, along with the cooked, shredded chicken you set aside. Turn off the heat when you add the chicken to prevent it from becoming tough. Leave to stand for 5 minutes, then serve in deep bowls with some soy or tamari sauce to taste. The noodles, greens and chicken are best eaten with chopsticks, but the soup is best drunk straight from the bowl.

- rapeseed oil
- flaxseed oil.

Bad fats
Saturated fats

Although many of these are found in 'natural' food, they do raise cholesterol and can be bad for you in excess; however, you should enjoy your food and have a little of what you fancy now and again. Saturated fats are found in:
- red meat, such as steak, high-fat mince, etc.
- egg yolks
- cheese
- coconut oil.

Trans fats

These are seriously bad for you and I recommend you avoid them. Trans fats are used to preserve foods for longer. They are found in:
- chips
- fried foods
- pre-packaged popcorn or popcorn made in the microwave
- some margarines.

Years ago, I read a book called *Fats That Heal, Fats That Kill: The Complete Guide To Fats, Oils, Cholesterol and Human Health* by Udo Erasmus, and this helped shape my thinking on fats. I was always a little sceptical of the idea that butter was so bad for you, especially when compared to some of the supposedly 'healthy' low-fat alternatives on the market. This book backed up my suspicions. I never eat margarine – it is made by a process known as hydrogenation, which uses the cheapest fats and mixes them together with metal particles. I view it as chemical muck and would urge you to bin it and treat yourself instead to the occasional teacake with butter.

So, a balanced diet means having a bit of the right fat. I still enjoy cooking my roast potatoes in goose fat (on the basis that olive oil should not be heated over 180°C). In her book *Nourishing Traditions*, Sally Fallon advocates putting a dollop of cultured cream into blended soup. She says: 'It supplies not only enzymes, but also valuable fat-soluble vitamins. These fat-soluble vitamins are what your body needs to utilize the minerals in the soup.'

Olive oil is great for use in salad dressings or drizzled over vegetables once roasted, and it can be used for cooking at a moderate heat.

Weight management issues
Undereating and binge eating (anorexia and bulimia)
Women with eating disorders such as anorexia nervosa or bulimia need to be treated by a psychiatrist before attempting to conceive. For further information on where to get help see *www.eating-disorders.org.uk* or *www.b-eat.co.uk*.

Overeating: fertility problems for the overweight and obese
In 1997, the medical journal the *Lancet* published research that suggested that the soaring levels of obesity in the West may trigger an infertility crisis among women in the next generation.[16]

Obesity goes hand in hand with fertility-related problems. Between a third and one half of women who have polycystic ovary syndrome (PCOS) are overweight or obese.[17] PCOS causes menstrual disorders, and considerable abnormal secretion of hormones, including those that control the reproductive cycle. The issue of weight can worsen what is already a tricky condition: 'In subfertile/infertile women with PCOS, overweight or obesity usually is more prevalent.'[18] But the good news is that overweight women who do lose weight bring their chances of conceiving both naturally and using fertility treatment, back in line with those who are not over-weight.

The central issues for those trying to lose weight are obviously diet and exercise. However, other essential tools that can help you to change bad habits are affirmation and self-hypnosis.

Studies show that you are more likely to lose weight successfully if you change your approach to food, rather than just reducing calories.[19] One of the most effective diets for those with PCOS is said to be the GI diet. The GI diet focuses on the glycaemic index, which measures the effects of carbohydrates on blood glucose levels. Those that are quickly broken down and released into the system are classed as having a 'high' GI, which are not as beneficial as those with a 'low GI'. The foods recommended in this diet all have a low glycaemic index (less than 55) and include:

- porridge, rice, bran, pasta, multi-grain bread, fruit loaf
- **most vegetables,** but *not* potatoes or sweet potatoes
- **legumes** – beans and lentils
- **fruit** – apples, grapes, orange, kiwi fruit. Some fruit is not 'low GI' (e.g. cantaloupe, honeydew and watermelon, raisins and dates), but may be recommended in the food groups for your type. Try to eat less of these where possible.

See Resources, page 360 for more information.

Chinese medicine and obesity

Chinese medicine sees obesity as an issue of Dampness (see page 116). It strongly cautions against attempts to lose weight by severely cutting back on food (which can weaken the spleen) or worse still, starvation.

I advise patients who are Damp and have weight issues to

steer clear of anything too cold, such as large quantities of cold water, raw foods and food straight from the fridge. In his book *Recipes for Self-Healing,* Daverick Leggett, author of several dietary books based on the principles of Chinese medicine, says: 'Overweight people need to nourish themselves rather than starve or punish themselves in order to regulate obesity. This means eating warm, cooked foods, plenty of vegetables soups and stews, a little lean and low-fat protein, whole grains and legumes, flavoured with gentle warm-energy pungent herbs and spices.' He goes on to warn that although sugar, saturated fat and refined starch need to be avoided, 'if over-restrictive, ultra-low calorie, Cold-energy diets are followed, the craving for those foods will simply increase.'[20]

In my practice, I suggest patients supplement their treatment with therapy to address underlying emotional issues because I find that those who work on their mental outlook and the way they view themselves have far more success battling weight issues than those who purely concentrate on diet. It is now fairly mainstream to tackle a serious weight problem as a symptom of other issues. Overeaters Anonymous have groups all over the country: *www.oagb.org.uk*

In Chinese medicine, working on your emotional relationship with food, is considered as important as diet and exercise. As Daverick Leggett, author of *Foods For Self Healing* says: 'Deeper at work in the psyche there are often powerful messages about the body that any amount of dieting will not shift.' He says that, once sensible eating measures have been introduced, patients need to learn a 'loving acceptance of the body'.[21]

For more information on how to confront issues of weight mentally, see the 'Is the mind on board?' sections throughout. The sections on affirmations and meridian tapping are particularly helpful. I strongly recommend daily morning affirmations, such as: 'As I attend to my emotional needs, my body rewards me by reducing in weight'; and 'My food choices are healthy and delicious and I feel deeply nourished and satisfied.'

How and what to drink
Water
Water has become a feature of many health fads in that people think they need to consume it in vast quantities, and

---

BODY MASS INDEX (BMI)

You may have heard about healthy weight in terms of a healthy body mass index (BMI). Body mass index is calculated as your weight (in kilograms) divided by your height (in metres) squared. For example, the average woman in the UK weighs 70 kilograms (11 stone) and is 1.61 metres (5 foot 3½ inches) tall, which means she has a BMI of 27.

$$\frac{BMI = weight}{(height \times height)} \quad \frac{BMI = 70}{(1.61 \times 1.61)} = 27$$

Here's how the scores are interpreted for adults:

Below 18.5:   *underweight*
18.5 – 24.9:   *healthy weight*
25 – 29.9:   *overweight*
30 and above: obese

Remember, though, that your BMI is just an indicator, not a cast-iron statement of fact. So if you're not sure whether or not you're overweight, it's best to check with your GP.

Women who are classified as 'overweight' or 'obese' (with a BMI of 25 or more) when they begin pregnancy are at a much higher risk of miscarriage, and have a greater risk of having high blood pressure, clots, diabetes and heart disease in pregnancy[22] They are also more prone to bleeding. As a result, there is also a greater risk of maternal death[23] among these women, as well as an increased risk of babies with birth defects[24] and stillbirth.[25] It is very important to correct your weight before you get pregnant. Being underweight (with a BMI of less than 18.5) is equally problematic in terms of fertility.

do so all day long, from large plastic bottles.

Water is important, yes (and particularly so during IVF). However, some types are misled into thinking they need to drink litres of it every day in order to stay 'healthy' and I see many patients who are stressed because they are not drinking their allocated 'three litres a day'. This is nonsense. Your fluid intake can come from a whole host of other sources like soups and teas. And not only is it unnecessary to drink copious amounts of water, it is also not particularly good for you.

A diet that is rich in nuts, berries and seeds (providing essential fatty acids and moisture) is what the body needs. And, of course, there are times when you'll need to increase your water intake: in very hot weather, when you are sweating or during a cycle of IVF. But generally speaking, your body should tell you if you are thirsty – you'll *feel* thirsty for a start, you may get headaches, dizzy spells and your urine will be darker.

In Chinese medicine, too much water interrupts the energy in the stomach and prevents it from properly performing its job of breaking down food, leaving it to sit in the bowel and ferment. Here are some tips for getting your fluid intake right:

- Don't drink while eating, it will flood your digestion and dilute digestive enzymes.
- Avoid 'dry' foods – many health foods, such as rice cakes and health bars, are extremely dry; no wonder you feel parched!
- The Chinese traditionally have a soup with every meal, which helps to increase their fluid intake (but watch out for salty soups).
- A cup of warm or room-temperature water with a slice of lemon followed by porridge will give you a good quota of fluid.

- Don't drink water from the fridge – drink warm water away from meals.

Coffee

Coffee receives a lot of flak, and I have to say that the coffee at the many chain stores across the country is pretty rancid. But one cup of good quality coffee a day, in the middle of the morning, does have things going for it. It stimulates the brain, the digestive system and the bowel and helps break down Stagnation and Dampness; however, it is *not* recommended for those who are Blood Deficient, Heat or Yin Deficient (see pages 121, 126 and 129).

Note: too much caffeine has been linked to early miscarriage, so please do limit your intake of any caffeinated drinks to one cup a day at most if you are trying to conceive.[26]

Tea

Herbal tea is an amazing drink and there are literally thousands of research papers demonstrating its health-giving properties, from protecting against cancer to lowering cholesterol. Instead of flooding the digestion with too much water or drinking coffee, try replacing it with some of the teas suggested below. It all counts as fluid and you have the added health benefits. Most of the teas I suggest are caffeine free or low in caffeine, which is preferable (see note on caffeine and miscarriage above).

The Chinese favour green tea, which I also love, but there are many different varieties of herbal tea to choose from and experiment with. Here are some of my favourites, but don't limit yourself, be adventurous:

- Green tea (which does contain caffeine)
- Chrysanthemum flower tea
- Nettle tea
- Raspberry leaf tea (but *not* in early pregnancy)

- Rosebud tea (*not* in pregnancy)
- Dandelion tea
- Ginger tea
- Chai

Milk

Some IVF units advise that patients drink large quantities of milk during their cycle. This is to make sure that they have enough protein in their diet. In Chinese medicine, however, milk is thought to create Dampness in the body, which, in the female reproductive system, can make women susceptible to the formation of cysts. These can disrupt the normal functioning of the menstrual cycle (see fertility types, page 108).

Daverick Leggett suggests warming milk with cardamom in order to make it easier to digest.[27] He also suggests separating meat from dairy because the acids produced by the stomach in order to digest meat are neutralized by milk. This, again, leads to Dampness.

Full-fat milk is often preferable to skimmed or semi-skimmed. As Leggett explains: 'The removal of fat to make low-fat milk is probably misguided. Removing the fat imbalances the food and increases the chances of adverse reactions in the body. When the level of fat is reduced the level of protein is relatively increased which in turn overtaxes the kidneys.'[28]

If you are asked by your IVF unit to increase your milk intake, consider instead consuming milk in its fermented form as yoghurt or crème fraîche, since the fermenting process breaks down the milk protein which is hard to digest; furthermore, some of the vitamin content will improve through fermenting.

Supplements

The UK Government recommends that pregnant women, and

anyone who is trying to conceive, should take a daily supplement of 400mcg of folic acid. There are also supplements targeted specifically at women trying to get pregnant. If you are concerned that you are not getting the requisite vitamins, minerals and oils, there is good reason to take supplements for fertility.

You need to ensure that you are taking, either in food or as a supplement, the recommended amounts of vitamins A, B1, B2, B5, B6, B12, C, folate, zinc, calcium, magnesium, selenium and essential fatty acids.

Sprouting

The Chinese have long used sprouting seeds and beans as a source of vitamin C, while sprouted mung beans were used by sailors in the eighteenth and nineteenth century on long ocean trips to prevent scurvy. Sprouted seeds and beans are delicious sprinkled on salads or added, right at the last minute, to soups.

The action of sprouting also increases vitamin D content, helps the absorption of calcium and the enzymes produced by sprouting aid the process of digestion. You can buy sprouting kits from any good health-food shop, and I recommend that you sprout your own (it can become quite a hobby) as they are often sold wrapped in cling film in the shops. It's one of life's little contradictions that the manufacturers understand the value of sprouting, but fail to grasp the harmful effects of cellophane.

Hazards: things to avoid
Alcohol

The ancient cities of Carthage and Sparta had laws banning newlyweds from drinking alcohol because a child conceived by intoxicated parents was thought to be unhealthy. Of course, 'intoxicated' is an extreme state, and many a healthy baby has been conceived after a couple of glasses of wine with dinner. And herein lies the point: alcohol, handled sensibly, actually has some health *benefits*.

Studies suggest that moderate drinkers are less likely to die from cardiovascular disease than non-drinkers, and have a reduced risk of developing Alzheimer's and other forms of dementia (drinkers of red wine, specifically). White wine, in moderation, is said to improve lung function, dark beer to prevent blood clotting and light beer to have possible benefits for cholesterol and antioxidant levels.[29]

FERMENTED FOODS

I spent much of my childhood in Germany because my father was posted there with the British Armed Forces. One of my abiding memories is of sauerkraut. My father disliked it, but we couldn't get enough of it!

Sauerkraut is made by fermenting cabbage. Including fermented foods in our diets today is good for our digestive systems because it replaces the lactobacilli in our gut (intestinal flora). The advent of pasteurization has meant that the practice of fermenting is dying out, but by simply including sauerkraut in your diet, you will increase your resistance to disease, make your bowel function better and improve your immune response. Cabbage is also great for the liver.

Sauerkraut

1 cabbage, finely chopped
1 tbsp caraway seeds
2 tbsps of good quality sea salt (such as Maldon)

1. Put the cabbage in a mixing bowl with the seeds and the salt and pummel with the end of a rolling pin until the cabbage starts to bleed its juices.

2. Pack the mixture into a freshly washed jam jar (or something similar), leaving a couple of centimetres free at the top.

3. Leave at room temperature for a few days, then store in the fridge. It will get better the longer you leave it.

ESSENTIAL FATTY ACIDS FOR FERTILITY

Essential fatty acids (EFAs) are *fatty* acids that cannot be produced in the body and which must, therefore, be obtained from the diet. They are generally divided into two groups – omega 3 and omega 6. Kate Cook, a specialist in nutrition for fertility,[30] says that it is vital to have a balance of these, and suggests the following:

- **For omega 6:** evening primrose oil and blackcurrant seed oil. Both of these reduce inflammation and enhance the release of sex hormones.[31] Blackcurrant seed oil also has a higher level of GLA (gamma-linolenic acid). You can also get omega 6 from nuts and seeds, legumes and certain vegetable oils, such as borage oil (but don't heat these). The recommended dose is two capsules, three times a day (Biotics 500mg oil, which provides 80mg GLA).
- **For omega 3:** this is found in oily fish. It is also good for inflammation and can be found in smaller amounts in walnuts and flax. Follow the recommended dose for supplements. Some oily fish contain pollutants, such as mercury; this is the case with tuna, which is only recommended once a week for pregnant women.

Unfortunately, the UK seems to be one of the last places on earth to grasp the concept of sensible drinking. Media reports show women 'intoxicated' in the extreme on high streets across the country. According to a report published by the National Health Service 16 per cent of women in the UK had 'hazardous' drinking patterns.[32]

Many women use pregnancy as the catalyst they need to give up drinking (and smoking), arguing that it's easier when you have the incentive actually growing inside you. Unfortunately, however, drinking and smoking can stand in the way of conception for many women, so that waiting until they conceive before quitting will not help them.

Alcohol affects both male and female fertility. In men, alcohol can affect sperm count and quality and can reduce the size of the testicles, leading to impotence, while in women, it interferes with hormones and affects the functioning of the menstrual cycle. The *British Medical Journal* showed that women who had as few as one to five glasses a week had decreased fecundability (the monthly probability of conception).

My rule of thumb with patients is that if they have any concerns about their drinking, they are probably drinking too much, and it's best to cut it out while trying to conceive. In my clinic, it's often (ironically) those who don't drink at all because of fears over fertility who could benefit from the very occasional glass of wine to help them relax.

How to drink alcohol

The one bit of advice my mother gave me, as I left home and headed for London, was: 'Don't drink the punch at parties'. In retrospect, this was sound advice. It's always a good idea to make sure you know exactly what you are drinking and in what quantities. Here are some ideas but, in general, you really should be thinking about absolute minimal alcohol intake:

- Never drink on an empty stomach – this is really important. The liver can process alcohol more efficiently if you have eaten.
- Alcohol is a hormone disruptor (affects the endocrine system), so if you suffer from thyroid problems, PCOS, endometriosis or PMT, you should limit alcohol intake or, if you are actively trying to conceive, think about avoiding it altogether.
- If you crave alcohol, you may find that eating carbohydrates – such as a plate of pasta – will help to combat the cravings.
- Milk thistle can help 'cleanse' the liver (see below).

Monosodium glutamate (MSG)

MSG has, for a long time, been used in Asian food. It is an artificial food additive and flavour enhancer which thickens food and sauces and has a starchy, faintly papery taste with a sharp aftertaste.

Studies have shown MSG to cause fertility problems in laboratory rats. Male rats fed MSG before mating had a less than 50 per cent success rate as opposed to 92 per cent in those that had not.

Q&A

How many units of alcohol can we drink while trying for a baby? Even moderate intake of alcohol in women can increase the time spent trying to conceive (4–7 units per week). For men I would suggest no more than 6 units. However for those patients who have Heat or Dampness (see Chapter Three) then alcohol needs to be strictly limited – and preferably avoided altogether.

Furthermore, the offspring from the rats fed MSG had shorter body length, reduced testes and tended to be overweight.[33]

Today, many products are advertised as MSG free, although this does not preclude any of the new generation of additives and enhancers. My advice is to cook fresh wherever possible, so that you know exactly what's in your food.

Other products that sometimes use MSG for bulk include stock cubes, packaged soups, tinned, prepared foods, seasoning mixtures, barbecue sauces, some soy sauces, salad dressings, some crisps, ready meals and processed and tinned meats.

Butylated hydroxyanisole (BHA)

BHA is thought to mimic oestrogens and interferes with the menstrual cycle, so should be avoided by fertility patients. It is used as a preservative and is added to a wide number of foods such as: butter, lard, meats, cereals, baked foods, sweets, beer, vegetable oils, snack foods, nuts and nut products, dehydrated potatoes and flavouring agents, sausages, poultry and meat products, dry mixes for drinks and puddings, glazed fruits, chewing gum, active dried yeast, defoaming agents for beet sugar and yeast, and emulsion stablizers for shortenings. Basically, always check the labels!

Other additives

Other additives to look out for in high quantities are:
- hydrolyzed protein (either vegetable or plant)
- hydrolyzed oat flour
- calcium caseinate
- sodium caseinate
- textured protein (including TVP)
- autolyzed yeast

Aspartame

Aspartame is an artificial sweetener or sugar substitute (common brand names include NutraSweet and Canderel). It is usually added to anything 'diet', such as fizzy drinks, as well as 'sugar-free' gums and breath fresheners. In Chinese medicine overconsumption of sweet substances, including artificial sweeteners and sugar, damages the digestion and leads to Dampness.

There has been much controversy over whether aspartame is safe, particularly in America, where some doctors have cited aspartame as a cause of infertility in animals. In a letter to the campaigning group Children of the New Earth, Dr Madelon Price states: 'I showed (in rodents) that both amino acids [aspartame and glutamate] freely enter the arcuate nucleus and (at low dose) cause inappropriate release of hormones and at high dose actually destroy these regulatory neurons. That is why sexual dysfunction is associated with aspartame and MSG. If enough arcuate neurons are lost, that dysfunction is irreversible. Rodents that ingest high levels of aspartate or glutamate when young become infertile adults.'[34]

Aspartame has also been implicated in miscarriage and a whole range of other health problems so my advice is straightforward: avoid it!

BE GOOD TO YOUR LIVER

- Eat plenty of green foods like seaweed, spinach and leafy greens.
- Start the day with a cup of hot water and a slice of lemon.
- Dandelion tea is a traditional liver remedy and will also help your digestion.
- Drink green tea – it contains catechins which help protect the liver.
- The plant milk thistle, which is available in tablet form, has been used for thousands of years to prevent damage and help repair the liver.
- Garlic is helpful to remove toxins from the body as well as improving immune function.
- Eat raw foods and vegetable juices, especially carrots and beetroot (but not for Cold or Damp types – see pages 112 and 116).
- Essential fatty acids in oily fish are also good for the liver.
- Lecithin supplements help to remove fat from the liver and lower cholesterol.

Smoking

The effects of smoking on fertility are well documented, but for anyone who hasn't been listening: smoking can have a catastrophic effect on the fertility of both women and men.

Smoking has been shown to have a negative impact both on conception – smokers take longer to conceive than non-smokers – and on the ability to carry a pregnancy to term. The risk of damaging fertility is only slightly smaller for passive smoking than it is for active smoking.

In men, smoking affects sperm count and the quality and motility of sperm. It causes a higher number of sperm with abnormal shape and function. In women, smoking can have an irreversible effect on the ovaries, accelerates the deterioration of eggs and can, in the long term, speed up the arrival of the menopause. Chemicals in cigarettes interfere with the production of oestrogen and the eggs of women who smoke have been shown to be more prone to genetic abnormality. Smoking is thought to cause an increased risk of miscarriage and of ectopic pregnancy. I urge you to go to the section on meridian tapping (pages 78–79) to help you quit.

Recreational drugs

Cocaine, marijuana, MDMA (Ecstasy) and any other recreational drug you care to mention have no place in a fertility programme – for either partner. These drugs will damage your chances of conceiving a baby in the first place, and pose a very serious threat to the development and health of any baby you do conceive.

If you are having trouble quitting, see on the section on meridian tapping in addition to seeking professional outside help. Check out www.talktofrank.com.

Is the mind on board?

Do not underestimate the power of your mind. If you can harness this power and make it work for you, almost anything is possible. I am going to give you the information you need to help you get your mind on side and working for you, to help you achieve a healthy pregnancy. I have seen with my own eyes that patients who work with their attitude and outlook can forge real changes at a deep level.

One of the biggest and most common problems is when your mind – consciously or unconsciously – decides to work against you. Outwardly, people may appear happy, balanced and self-confident, while inwardly they are gripped by a tempest from the second they wake up in the morning. In my experience, some people become adept at hiding their inner turmoil in order to succeed in life, and it is often these people who find that churned-up, yet buried emotions start to affect their health and ability to conceive. (For more on this, see Chapter Two on self-assessment.)

In Chinese medicine, the heart is directly linked to the womb and each can impact on the other. Each of us needs to work through our emotional issues so that they don't hold us back. When they are too big to deal with alone, it's best to work through them with a professional.

There are a number of techniques you can use to deal with emotional issues that may be standing in the way of your fertility health. Below, is everything that my patients have used to achieve positive outcomes. This includes the template for some groundbreaking work I have done with Emma Roberts on meridian tapping which, although a new, and at the time of writing, clinically untested technique, has produced truly amazing results – particularly for IVF.

Happiness

We all live in the pursuit of happiness, that elusive state of contentment, of heightened joy, untarnished by worry. For some people, happiness is uproarious laughter, while for others it's just feeling mellow. You may experience it relaxing in the bath, surrounded by candles, on a country walk on a summer's evening or enjoying the company of friends over a delicious home-cooked supper.

The actual act of laughter is incredibly therapeutic. Studies show that laughing actually promotes vasodilation – the widening of blood vessels – which, in turn, relaxes the muscles and lowers blood pressure.[35] I know a patient who saves up comedy programmes to watch in the last two days of her cycle – a time when she used to rage uncontrollably.

Feelings of happiness have almost immediate effects on the immune system. Peter Deadman, editor of the *Journal of Chinese Medicine*, says: 'Within twenty minutes of happy thoughts being experienced, the amount of antibody immuno-globulin (sIgA) found in the saliva doubles, remaining raised for at least three hours.'[36] See? Happiness is healthy.

Unfortunately, however, even when we do experience it, happiness is often transient. As Peter Deadman writes: '[The] memory of [a] traumatic or painful experience causes the sIgA levels to drop.'[37] Once happiness is gone we stress and fret about getting back to that relaxed, balanced state.

My own view is that we all need to deal with the negative emotions in our lives, and either get rid of them or turn them into positives. Remember: it's not what happens to you in life, it's the way you deal with it. In Chinese medicine, working through the issues that hold you back is called cultivation of the mind. A similar concept in Western medicine is cognitive behavioural therapy (CBT).

You can cultivate your mind through meditation. Some people wave this away and saying, it's too difficult. But don't be put off. See my section below on meditation.

Peter Deadman says: 'There is ample evidence that avoiding intense negative emotions, calming the mind, laughing, being in intimate relationships with others and cultivating generosity, all contribute to good health and longevity.'[38] On the flip side, bad habits can lead to behavioural patterns that ultimately result in us becoming unhappy and 'stagnated' – a frame of mind that we all want to avoid in life, but particularly patients who are trying to conceive.

Stop complaining

Are you a moaning Minnie? One of the most common negative traps you can fall into is that of complaining. It is both addictive and catching. Anyone who has ever worked in an office knows how easy it is to get dragged into the downward spiral of complaining about the boss, the hours, the workload and so on.

When you complain you see things through a negative filter. Often, the reason is that you are frustrated, and complaining somehow makes you feel as if you are 'getting things off your chest'. In Chinese medicine, this is a classic symptom of Qi stagnation. You may feel momentarily better for airing your grievance, but it is not a long-lasting solution. Complaining doesn't relieve you of the frustration, it only serves to grind you further into a rut.

Try a little mental exercise. Every time you are about to complain, stop yourself, take a deep breath and say something positive instead. Gradually, over the course of a day, you will be amazed by how much better you feel. If you are in a particularly moany office environment, try to distract someone else who is complaining with a positive thought or conversation topic. Or make them laugh. (There are, of course, terminal complainers who are impossible to distract and in such cases you may have to limit the amount of time you spend with them – tactfully.)

Positive thinking

Every night as he tucked me into bed, my father used to say to me: 'Every day in every way, it's getting better and better.' This little phrase set me up for a lifetime of positive thinking – what a gift.

Back in the 1970s when I was small, we didn't know what science has taught us today: that the mind really can impact the body at a cellular level. And plenty of people today still don't believe in optimism. They think it is just a state of mind that briefly boosts morale so that we can continue toiling through our pointless existence. But as well as boosting morale, optimism also boosts our ability to achieve positive outcomes.

In 2007, a study at the University of Toledo, Ohio tested the theory that optimists and pessimists could, to some extent, control the outcome of their medical treatment. First, both groups were given a placebo and told that they would experience negative side effects. The pessimists felt far worse than the optimists. Then, researchers gave both groups a sleep treatment – again a placebo – telling them that it would encourage good sleep. The optimists enjoyed far better sleep than the pessimists. The conclusion was, of course, that optimists respond well to treatment that they believe may help them.[39] As David Hamilton, author of *How Your Mind Can Heal Your Body,* says: 'The key to healing lies within us.'[40]

Affirmations will help you believe in your goal, as will meditation (see pages 72 and 76). Ask yourself while you are meditating what it is that you need to feel better. Sometimes, when you are in a place of quiet contemplation, you can find that you have all the answers within you. Have confidence in your own abilities to overcome any obstacles. I like the Winston Churchill quote: 'The pessimist sees the difficulty in every opportunity; an optimist sees the opportunity in every difficulty.'

Comparing yourself with others

Another truly human and very self-destructive trait is the desire to compare ourselves to others. We are all, by our nature and upbringing, pretty competitive beings – something that is evident in children and in adults.

I see some women for whom fierce competition and the drive to compare themselves with their peers is a real obstacle in their approach to fertility. They have learnt to compete on every level, whether it's about acquiring possessions or rising up the ranks in a competitive workplace.

An oft-quoted survey carried out in 1985 found that levels of happiness and wellbeing experienced by those featured in the Forbes List of the 400 wealthiest Americans were equal to those of the Masai, the traditional herdsmen of East Africa, who are at the opposite end of the financial spectrum.[41] It is, ultimately, your outlook that makes for the best form of happiness, i.e. long-term happiness.

Some women set out to conceive because they think that's what they ought to be doing at a given point in time – that it is expected of them. They are pursuing a 'goal' for all the wrong reasons. And then, when they can't conceive, the immediate effect is devastating. All their friends are conceiving, having baby showers, giving birth, then hanging out together doing 'play dates'. That can make them feel anxious and knotted-up inside and, in some cases, they feel they have failed and are bitter towards their friends. It's all completely understandable. But these negative feelings can stagnate and create, in turn, a negative cycle of thoughts. They can also create anger and resentment. I do a lot of work in this area, and seeing people let go of these long-held, disruptive attitudes is very rewarding because it is life-changing for them: it brings long-term happiness.

It's important to learn to let go of general comparisons with others when it comes to fertility. When the genes were handed out, some people did better than others. The Chinese call the constitution we are all born with our Jing, and while there is nothing we can do to change this, we can optimize what we have by living to the best of our own limits.

One mental exercise I get my patients to do is to imagine that they are holding their baby in their arms, surrounded by their friends who also have children. If you positively visualize your baby it can have a very calming effect. Perhaps try this together with some affirmations: 'I am preparing my body for a very healthy conception, so that one day I can hold my healthy, gorgeous baby in my arms.'

Appreciate what you have

This is another way to train your mind to concentrate on the positive. Try spending five to ten minutes of every day scribbling down all the things in your life that you are grateful for and happy about. It might be friends or relationships, or a warm exchange you had with a colleague that day. When you find yourself feeling hard-done by or frustrated, or when you start comparing yourself to others, this simple little exercise may help you feel more upbeat and positive about yourself.

The power of affirmations

Many of the negative thoughts that revolve around our brains on a loop have been there for a long time – since childhood, even. The point here is to reset that loop with positive thoughts.

Affirmations can help you to focus in on what you are trying to achieve or bring into your life. They are positive statements of fact. They are intentions: statements that you wish to be true, to become fact. You have to repeat them in order to reinforce the desire.

The first time you attempt affirmations, you may feel self-conscious and a little silly. This is why it's so important to try them on a daily basis, so that you stop feeling this way. You can do affirmations with or without visualizations (see page 75), but the most important thing is that you repeat them as often as possible, because the more times you repeat something, the greater the connection it makes in the brain.

David Hamilton writes: 'Repeating a statement about something being true will create neural connections as though we were experiencing the thing being true and were making a statement of fact.'[42] Here are some examples:

- 'My ovaries are healthy and work perfectly, releasing an egg every month.'
- 'I will become pregnant when my body is ready and I am healthy and well.'
- 'My relationship is good and I feel supported.'

Make your affirmations as brave and bold as you feel:

- 'This is a new day and a new opportunity to get healthy and fit for conception.'
- 'I am going to embrace each step of this journey because it is an investment in my health and happiness, and in the health of my baby.'
- 'I love myself, I respect myself and I can let go of the things that hold me back in my path towards a healthy conception.'
- 'I feel free and relaxed and happy. I am me; I am happy with me.'
- 'I am better NOW!'

I tell my patients that rather than seeing the arrival of their period as a sign of failure, they should tell themselves: 'This gives me another month in which I can prepare my body to be healthy and fertile.'

If a patient is ruminating all day long about falling pregnant I try to get them to be disciplined, by setting time aside in the day for some mindful practice towards their goal, rather than letting their minds wander to it and invade their thinking. Ten minutes at either end of the day is good.

Some people do prefer to go with their mind when it wanders, which is also fine, but make sure that yours is working for you rather than against you. So many people sabotage their own efforts by having no faith in themselves. You *can* achieve this. You *can* change your life; you are doing it right now – it's a choice. Simply do the affirmations as often as you need to in order to feel good about yourself.

It takes practice to turn negative thought patterns into positive ones, but it is effective. I've seen countless patients who have told themselves that something negative is true so many times that they have *made* it true. Often, this is about their fertility: they start out believing they *may* have an issue conceiving, and this then manifests as an actual physical problem that blocks conception.

You need to turn these thoughts around. Train yourself to think positive thoughts about your health and fertility. Concentrate on the area that needs healing. As the saying goes: 'Energy flows where the attention goes.'

There have been many studies into the power of mind over matter, but one that I particularly like looked at building up the muscles in the finger. The volunteers were divided into two groups. The first group actually did finger exercises, while the second *imagined* they were doing the finger exercises. In each training session, the groups did fifteen real or imagined contractions at a time followed by a twenty-second rest period, five days a week for twelve weeks. At the end of the three months, the muscle strength of both groups was tested.

In the first group, muscle strength had improved by 53 per

cent, while in the second group – those who had done nothing but imagine the exercises – it had improved by 35 per cent, even though they hadn't lifted a finger (literally).[43]

Your brain can generate a physical response to something that you concentrate on in the mind – whether this is negative or positive.

Visualization

Visualization has become increasingly popular in all areas of healthcare – and I'm not surprised. It is *so* effective. There are many ways of using visualization. In labour, for instance, it is often used as a tool to distract from the pain – for example by seeing the contraction as a wave crashing against the shore – and turn it into a more tangible idea. In my work, it is useful for helping women to 'see' what is happening inside their bodies, and to direct its course in order to achieve the outcome they desire.

For example, if I have a patient who is not ovulating I get them to imagine strongly the process of reproduction from Day 1 of their cycle, concentrating on the mechanics of ovulation around Day 14. It may sound nuts, but when combined with acupuncture it really can work (see Case Study on page 207).

When you start tracking your menstrual cycle, spend a few minutes every day visualizing what is happening in your womb (see Chapter Four for a detailed description of the reproductive process). The best way to practise this is in a calm, quiet environment, where you are relaxed and alone, without interruptions. I like to do it sitting cross-legged, with my shoulders relaxed and my hands resting gently on my knees. You can use this position or any that you find comfortable.

Self-hypnosis

If you have been visualizing and repeating your affirmations, you are already in the zone of self-hypnosis. A further step you may want to take is to create your own tape of lovely, soft affirmations that you can listen to as you relax.

When you relax, really think about the actual process of relaxing. Talk yourself into a state of deep relaxation on the tape which you can lie down on your bed and listen to. Don't worry about falling asleep – the affirmations will still enter

MEDITATION

Meditation is used in many different cultures and is a powerful tool for achieving inner calm. For the purposes of this book we are going to touch on the basics of meditation. To find out more about the art of meditation, such as that practised by Buddhist monks, you can visit *www.how-to-meditate. org*. Monks believe that because the stresses we experience come from our mind, the practice of quietening the mind helps us achieve inner peace and contentment.

As with visualizations, you need to find somewhere quiet to practise. You can adopt the cross-legged yogi position if you find it comfortable, or just sit, with your back straight and your eyes gently closed.

The idea is that you are going to clear your mind and this can be hard for those with busy, hectic lives. Each time a thought comes into your mind, however, let it drift out again, like a cloud. It is often the case that when you start practising you find your mind getting busier with thoughts and ideas, but part of learning how to meditate is getting into the habit of gently batting these thoughts away.

Breathe through your nostrils, focusing on the way your health enters and leaves your body. Concentrate on this alone. Let your breathing be natural and unforced. The idea is to allow your mind to become still by concentrating on your even breathing. This in itself is a discipline. If you do this regularly it will become easier and you will become calmer. I recommend you try it once a day for 15 minutes, increasing your practice as you become better at it.

Meditating on your breath is, of course, just the first step in meditation. But you will find it is enormously rewarding. You will feel less stressed overall, your relationships will improve, as will your overall health.

your subconscious.

Try saying something along these lines:

- Relax your toes, then your feet.
- Think about your heels sinking into the bed.
- Relax your lower legs, concentrate on letting the calf muscles go.
- Relax your knees.
- Relax your thighs and feel your entire leg sinking deep into the bed.
- Continue up, thinking about your stomach and chest, then your fingers, hands, arms and – importantly – your shoulders.
- Let your shoulders drop right down; consciously feel the tension dropping out of them.
- Feel the sinking sensation in your entire body. Imagine you are sinking into soft grass and making an imprint in the earth below.
- Relax your neck, your jaw, your face, your mouth, cheeks, eyes, the area around the eyes and your forehead.
- Perhaps imagine roots growing from your body and pulling you into the earth beneath you. You are sinking deeper and deeper.
- Allow your mind, and your mind alone, to drift for a while until you feel as if it is floating above the physical you. As your mind floats, conjure up an image of yourself walking down three steps, slowly, step by step, feeling each step as you take it, until you are in a beautiful room where you feel happy and comfortable. Sit down on a huge comfortable chair and relax.

The aim of this exercise is to achieve a state of total and complete relaxation. You can embellish this basic structure as much as you like, but the winding-down process needs to be slow-paced. Once you have done that, you can start taping your own personal visualizations and/or your affirmations too.

You could visualize an issue being resolved inside your body, you could visualize conception, being pregnant, holding your baby or even being surrounded by an entire family of loved ones. If that feels too painful or difficult to imagine, visualize yourself taking the steps you need to take to obtain your goal. Remind yourself how happy and relaxed you are. You could also visualize letting go of problems – one tried-and-tested method is to imagine putting all your problems in a box, then flinging it out of a window where it will hit some imaginary rocks far below, breaking into pieces finer than dust.

Play about with ideas and see what works for you. If you think your tape is too personal for your partner to hear, try using headphones. Some patients say that making the tape to music and using their softest, kindest, calmest voice is effective.

If you don't want to make your own tape, you can download one from the Internet. There are many sites worth looking at; see Resources.

Supporting therapies

Supporting therapies are the techniques that I regularly use in the clinic to support the baby-making plan.

Meridian tapping

Meridian tapping is an extraordinarily effective and increasingly popular technique derived from acupuncture. I now see 'tapping' on television, whether it's for tennis players between sets or athletes as they limber up for a race.

The tapping techniques I discuss in this book were devised together with Emma Roberts, and Sue Beer, who are both clinical hypnotherapists, NLP Practitioners (neurolinguistic programming psychological therapy), and EFT Masters (Emotional Freedom Technique is the name given to meridian tapping by Gary Craig, the American founder), and are early pioneers of the tapping technique in this country.[44]

Meridian tapping is a way to free ourselves from the ongoing emotional and physical damage caused by traumas we have experienced. It uses the same energy points – or meridians – as acupuncture, and the gentle tapping of these points clears energy blockages that obstruct our efforts to achieve our goals. The idea is that tapping sends a vibration along the body's energy meridian, and if you focus simultaneously on a specific emotional issue, the tapping vibrations will cause the corresponding emotional blockage to shift.

For the purposes of this book, use of meridian tapping is limited to the IVF chapter (see page 320), but it does have many other fantastic applications, including helping with addiction – such as quitting smoking – overcoming a childhood trauma and losing weight.

Acupuncture

Acupuncture works on the principle that the body's optimum function is achieved when there is a balanced flow of energy, or Qi, along the meridian points of the body. This energy can be put out of balance, or disturbed, by any number of factors – including illness, stress, emotional trauma, bad diet and even the weather – and that in turn can affect physical health.

Among other things, channels can be 'blocked' and your Qi can become depleted, which can, in turn, cause heath issues, such as infertility. One explanation for how acupuncture might work is that when we stimulate acupuncture points we stimulate the pituitary gland which directly affects the function of the ovaries, adrenal and thyroid. There is evidence that by needling the body more beta-endorphins are released and this may encourage the body's innate healing process; it certainly makes the recipient feel good. In my experience, acupuncture appears to have a regulating effect on women's hormones and changes in the menstrual cycle can often be noted within one or two menstrual cycles.

Acupuncture has been the subject of a range of clinical studies to Western standards in Western medical settings. These tend to compare the results of groups of people who have received acupuncture with those who haven't. Some studies use 'sham acupuncture' to create a placebo. It has had proven results as a treatment for pain relief,[45] symptoms of the menopause,[46] post-operative nausea,[47] to name a few. It is also a popular treatment for insomnia, depression, addiction and common medical complaints such as colds, flu and sinusitis.

Another area of success for acupuncture is, of course, in the treatment of fertility. In 2008, the *British Medical Journal* published a groundbreaking review of seven carefully selected studies undertaken in Western countries, which found that women who had acupuncture were 65 per cent more likely to go on to have a successful embryo transfer procedure and 91 per cent more likely to have a live birth.[48]

Acupuncture must be done by a trained and recognized practitioner – if in doubt, check.[49] However, acupressure – applying steady pressure to acupuncture points with the fingers – is a technique that you can do yourself at home.[50] I know many women who have used acupressure during their menstrual cycle and I suggest various points for you to try throughout the book.

Moxibustion and warming techniques

These techniques are used to warm the body in the case of Cold, Cold/Damp and Yang Deficient (see pages 112, 116 and 131), especially when the lower abdomen is cold to touch.

In moxibustion, a herbal stick (moxa) is lit and held over

acupuncture points or areas of the body in order to warm and activate them. I use it when the lower abdomen is cold, on points like ST36 to energize the body (see diagram on page 125), Moxa is a good treatment to use when there is too much cold and for Yang-Deficient types or sometimes we use it to increase blood flow to the area.

In clinic, I often put moxa directly on to the needle, which is known as 'hot needle technique'; it is a wonderfully restorative treatment and works at a deep level to build the reproductive Qi. I also give patients a 'Womb Warmer' to use at home; this is a small heat pad that can be placed on the lower abdomen and used again and again. (See Resources for information on moxibustion equipment suppliers.)

Electroacupuncture

In this technique, needles are inserted into acupuncture points, then clips are attached and a small current is passed through them. Patients experience a not unpleasant vibration at the meridian points.

I use electroacupuncture to improve pelvic blood flow, thicken the endometrium and to stimulate the ovaries. I find that patients feel very 'floaty' after this treatment and deeply relaxed, which I put down to the endorphin release.

Auricular acupuncture

This involves the placing of small needles on points in the ear.

In my clinic, I use auricular acupuncture as part of normal practice. It is particularly useful for work with addictions and during IVF. It involves the insertion of tiny needles into the ear. Patients really enjoy auricular acupuncture, and it seems to promote the release of endorphins.

Herbal medicine

It is estimated that the Chinese herbalist has the choice of some five thousand substances to work with, and more than 100,000 different herbal prescriptions have been tested over the centuries.[51]

Over hundreds of years, doctors of Chinese medicine have compiled meticulous records about the plants and herbs they use, placing great emphasis on the safety of the patient. In the UK, we are learning more and more about these herbs and the Register of Chinese Herbal Medicine (RCHM) works with

TIPS FOR USING MOXA

Moxa is a plant (Artemisia argyi Folium) that is used as a heat source to stimulate acupuncture points and is easy to use yourself at home. You can buy a traditional variety or a smokeless variety in the form of a cigar-like 'stick' from Chinese medicine shops. I prefer the traditional ones, but they are incredibly smoky and many people can not tolerate them. If you do go for this variety you may need to use it with all the windows open.

Before using moxa you will need to prepare the following: a cigarette lighter or matches, a small ashtray to tap the ash into, a small towel to protect any fabric near where you are using the stick and a glass screw-top jar in which to put out the moxa stick at the end of the treatment.

To use

- Light one end of the moxa stick. Hold the lit end two to three centimetres from the back of your hand and feel the warmth.
- Hold the lit end of the stick over the area to be treated. Always keep the stick two to three centimetres away from you and never make direct contact with the skin.
- Acupuncture points can be warmed with the moxa stick for five to seven minutes over each point or until the area begins to feel hot.
- Any ash that forms on the end of the stick can be gently brushed off by using the edge of the ashtray
- Never touch the lit end of the moxa stick even if it looks like it has gone out.
- When you have finished, extinguish the stick by putting it lit-end down in your jar and putting the lid on.

the Bristol Chinese Herb Garden and the Royal Botanic Gardens, Kew, in building botanical knowledge of high-quality herbal medicines.

Chinese herbs are very safe when prescribed correctly by a properly trained practitioner; always check that you are seeing someone who is recognized by the RCHM. Adverse reactions can occur with all medicines, but they are rare in Chinese medicine. If you have any concerns, contact the RCHM (see Resources).

Aromatherapy

Aromatherapy is the use of essential oils as a natural remedy. Essential oils are diluted in a base oil, such as almond oil, They can be burnt, used in the bath or to enhance treatments such as massage. Some oils are contraindicated in pregnancy, so it is worth checking anything you use first. For more information on the use of essential oils, contact Neals Yard (see Resources).

Yoga

Some years ago I asked my colleague Uma Dinsmore-Tuli to develop a yoga practice that would work to optimize each phase of the menstrual cycle and would help harmonise the natural rhythms of the body. In this way, I felt patients could do something proactive between acupuncture treatments to enhance its effects. I explained to Uma what was happening energetically in the body from a Chinese medicine point of view and asked her to study the body's physical requirements at each phase. With this in mind, she has created a yoga sequence for fertility, which you will find in Appendix I (see page 334).

Yoga is an ancient practice that understands the body's energy flow and how the mind can influence the body. It is because of this that I think it is an ideal form of exercise for women who are trying to conceive. I really believe that if you are trying to get pregnant then you need to honour your body's needs and work with what nature has given you. The aim of the yoga in this book is to be a supportive and nourishing practice which adapts to meet your needs rather than force the body and work against the goal of conception. For this reason the sequences suggested have been designed to work in tandem for your particular requirements at any given phase of the menstrual cycle and to support the other suggestions given in this book.

Next steps

The first thing I do with my fertility patients is a 360-degree diagnosis. I am handing that over to you in the next chapter.

Chapter Two

The 360-degree health check

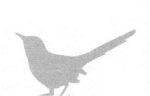

When a couple first arrive in my clinic, I always start with what I call the 360-degree health check. The aim of this 'fertility self-assessment' is to get your body and mind completely in balance and to be in the best possible health for conception. This check comprises questions about all aspects of your health and covers the same themes as in Chapter One: Is the engine working? Is the fuel good? Is the mind on board?

Keep in mind your goal of a healthy conception and a healthy baby at all times. You are about to embark on an exciting journey.

Trying to achieve balance

We will look at a whole range of 'symptoms', from the colour of your tongue to the length of your menstrual cycle, to work out if your body is showing signs of being out of balance. It may be that your system is showing a tendency towards what Chinese medicine terms as Cold, in which case we'd need to rebalance this with some warmth, using exercise, diet and changes to our environment. You will start to build a picture of what 'type' you are, which will enable you to start to make positive changes.

Everyone needs a little adjustment here and there, some more than others. I call it 'fine-tuning the engine'. Most people also find that they identify with more than one tendency. So, you may find yourself agreeing with statements that correspond to 'Qi Stagnation' as well as to Cold. This might be more apparent when you start to look at 'emotional'

GROWING A HEALTHY BABY

The idea of a 'baby-making' plan may seem unnecessary, particularly if you haven't yet met with any problems conceiving. However, I strongly believe that the healthier you are when you conceive, the healthier your conception and pregnancy will be. And you also pass the gift of health on to the next generation.

I ask my patients – both those who are receiving fertility treatment and those who are not – to think about it like this: imagine you have been to a garden centre and have found an exquisite, beautiful and rare plant. You excitedly rush home to put it in the soil where it will grow. But there is a problem: you have forgotten to weed the soil first. There is an area that is waterlogged and, actually, the soil is not as good as it could be. To put this treasured plant in

such sub-standard soil would be foolish. The plant will struggle to thrive without the correct environment and balance of nutrients. You could add a bit of fertilizer in the hope that this will make up for all the shortcomings, but in your heart you know that your plant deserves better.

The plant is symbolic of the egg, of course. And the soil is your womb. You want to conceive, but you also want to conceive in the best, most fertile soil. Your body needs to look after, nurture and nourish that egg for nine months as it develops from its embryonic stages into your beautiful baby.

Patients find that following my plan helped them to prepare for the extraordinary journey of pregnancy and parenthood.

symptoms in addition to the physical ones. If this is the case, read the advice for both and work with the type that you most closely identify with at any one time.

You may also find that your type changes or that you develop symptoms of one type even briefly. For example: if you spend a day exposed to powerful air conditioning, you may start showing symptoms of Cold. If you treat these symptoms, you will rebalance quickly. Try not to get too hung up on the diagrams, rather focus on the most obvious symptoms.

There may be times when you might find all this too difficult or a bit strange. All I can say is: please trust me. If you can begin to think about your body and your health in a new way, and start to take steps to improve and balance them, you will begin to become more aware of your body and how it works and what can affect it – both positively and negatively. The things I will teach you will take you closer to your goal of having a healthy conception and a healthy baby; I know it works for my patients, and it can work for you too.

Because we are working with the menstrual cycle, most of this advice is aimed at women. However, I have also included a male cycle on page 196 and a box on how to create healthy sperm on page 46.

What are the fertility types?
....

In this chapter and the next chapter I am going to refer to the following 'types':
- Cold
- Damp
- Blood Deficient
- Stagnant (which is separated into Liver Qi – or Qi Stagnant – and Blood)
- Heat

Q&A

My parents had me when they were both in their 40s; will this affect my fertility?
It would depend on their overall health. As a general rule, children born to older parents inherit poorer Jing. But if they were in very good health and your mother took care of herself while pregnant then this would have a positive effect on your health. If they were in poor health then the Jing may not be so abundant.

You can also have combined conditions, for example: Damp/Heat or Cold/Damp. You could also have Damp/Heat leading to Blood Deficient. I also use a number of key Chinese medicine terms:

- **Qi** – Your vital life force, the energy that circulates within the meridians, the motivating force behind all your bodily functions. This is explained more fully on page 89.
- **Qi** – Deficient Overall vitality is not as it could be; vital energy is lacking.
- **Jing** – The energy that you inherit from your parents; your constitution (your genetic predisposition). Your Jing declines with age and is a direct reflection on your reproductive capacity.
- **Shen spirit;** – Your spark for life. This is responsible for feelings of contentment, stability and a sense of being engaged and connected to life. It plays a big part in ovulation. When I talk about 'getting the mind on board', I am working on the shen.
- **Yin and Yang** – The iconic 'yin yang' symbol represents the two opposing yet interdependent energies: Yin is cool and nourishing and calming, whereas Yang is active, motivating and warm. You will learn that Yin represents the beginning part of your menstrual cycle – the stage where you grow follicles – and Yang takes over in the second phase, when you become a human incubator for the fertilized egg.
- **Meridians** – There are twelve main meridians, each one pertaining to an organ system. All along these meridians are acupuncture points, a few of which I will teach you to use yourself.

Identifying your chief symptom

Shortly after walking through the door and hanging up their coats, my patients explain their exact reason for coming to see me. In the vast majority of cases, it is a physical complaint. Western medicine calls this: 'the chief symptom', and it could be anything from, 'I have been trying to conceive for eight months – can you help?' to 'I haven't had a period for two years – why?'

Western medicine will treat ten patients with the same symptom in the same way. Chinese medicine, however, treats the whole person, so that no two patients will leave with the same treatment.

I want you to write down your chief symptom at the top of a blank page. Then write down your answers to the statements below. This will help you determine your type and to decide which course of action to follow in Chapter Four.

Should you discover unanticipated obstacles in your fertility journey that need input from other medical professionals in addition to this book, Part Three (see pages 243–330) guides you through the tests associated with fertility issues and, if necessary, fertility treatment.

Qi

After I have established why the patient has come to my clinic, I will begin taking notes on the overall quality of their Qi (see above).

If you have great Qi, you might be bouncing out of bed in the morning, taking a light jog to work and waving a cheery hello to your neighbours as you go; if you have depleted Qi, however, you might peer over the duvet with one eye, hoping that you still have another hour of sleep ahead of you.

Your Qi will be evident in your:
- overall energy
- demeanour
- voice
- complexion.

Questions to ask yourself are:
- Do I get ill often?
- Am I frequently tired?
- Do I find it hard to recover from illness?
- Am I the first to leave a party?
- Do I find it hard to get out of bed in the morning?
- Do I have a 'quiet' or 'thin' voice?
- Does my skin look tired?

If you answer 'Yes' to more than four of the above, you are exhibiting some tell-tale signs of a depleted Qi – a sort of less-than-best vitality. But don't worry. Modern life depletes Qi and it's a common issue – one I work with every day. This book will help you turn your Qi into a veritable force to be reckoned with.

How can I cultivate good Qi?

The approach to cultivating good Qi needs to be gentle and enjoyable – it shouldn't feel like you are being punished. As a general guideline you should aim to:
- eat well – according to your type
- balance your emotions and get the mind on board
- live according to your individual constitution (Jing) – by which I mean understand your strengths and weaknesses; don't compare yourself to others
- balance your working life and the rest of your life; neither over- nor underwork
- keep the engine well oiled – exercise, practise yoga or

qigong (these two forms of exercise actually generate Qi within the body).

Your menstrual cycle

Obviously, your menstrual cycle is your reproductive system and in Chapters Four to Seven we will go through the cycle in detail, working on optimizing each of the four parts of the cycle to get you in fantastic health to conceive.

It is said that a good practitioner of Chinese medicine can tell everything about a woman's health from her menstrual symptoms alone. The menstrual cycle dictates almost everything it is to be 'female' in both Western and Chinese medicine. The hormones that facilitate the cycle, like a wheel kept in motion by water, determine your mood, the way you look, feel, behave and even the way you dress.

Fertility patients, more than anyone else, need to be in tune with their menstrual cycle. They need to know what is in the realms of normal and what is not.

Length of cycle

To calculate the number of days of your cycle, count as Day 1 the first day of your period. Stop counting the day before your next period. Anything between twenty-seven and thirty-one days long is normal.

Travel, emotional stress and illness can

Qi-Building Flapjacks

The molasses, dates and oats in this recipe are invigorating to the Qi, while the butter is good for blood circulation. It is important when taking care of your pre-conceptual nutrition to remember to nourish your naughty side. A world with sweetness is a happy one.

230g butter
115g blackstrap molasses
115g cooked dates mashed to a paste (add a little water if too thick)
115g chopped cherries and/or coconut
340g oats
cinnamon, to taste

Melt the butter, molasses and mashed dates until creamy and thick. Add the chopped cherries/coconut, then fold in the oats and cinnamon. Bake in a rectangular tin (approx. 29cm by 19cm) at 180°C for 20 minutes. Cut into squares and serve.

all alter the length of the menstrual cycle, so factor in any major disruptions. Perhaps take the mean number of your last five cycles to get a good idea.

Longer and shorter cycles

If your cycle is regularly between twenty-one and twenty-six days, it may be that you are 'Qi Deficient'. Everyone is susceptible to Qi Deficiency at some point in their life, which is why it is not a stand-alone 'type' in this book. You may have a lot of what Chinese medicine calls Heat in your system. On the other hand, a cycle that is regularly thirty days long may indicate too much Cold in the system.

If your cycle is always irregular and difficult to chart, you may be experiencing a combination of Qi Stagnation and Blood Stagnation. Make a note of this and compare it with other symptoms. You will probably find that you are strongly emerging as a particular 'type' as you read through the rest of this chapter.

Your period

Do you have heavy periods? In other words, does your period either last a long time or do you lose a lot of blood? Either way this can indicate weak Qi or Heat.

Do you have scant periods? This means that either your periods are short or that there is only a little blood. It signals Blood Deficiency.

Have you stopped having periods? This is known as amenorrhoea and, again, this can be a sign of severe Blood Deficiency and Cold.

If you have never had a period, I would recommend that you ask your GP to refer you to a gynaecologist, in addition to following the advice in this book.

Blood loss

The amount of blood loss can vary, but the average is 30–80ml (and no, I don't expect you to measure this!).

Colour

Menstrual blood is dark red. On Day 1 the colour is a little lighter and becomes darker after a couple of days before turning a pinky colour towards the end. However, if your menstrual blood is closer to one of the descriptions below, you need to work on rebalancing it:

- Bright red, like a postbox – Heat
- Dark – Cold
- Purple – Cold
- Brown – also indicates Cold
- Pale – Blood Deficient
- Blackish – Blood Stagnation

Consistency

Menstrual blood should flow evenly with the greatest blood loss taking place within the first twenty-four hours. It shouldn't be too thick or too watery. It should be without clots.

- Watery – Blood Deficient
- Large clots – Blood Stagnation
- Small clots – Cold
- Clotted with fresh clots – Heat
- Clotted with older-looking clots –Blood Stagnation *and* Cold

Pain

Brace yourself for a controversial statement: your period should not be accompanied by pain. We have for so long associated periods with pain that it is now widely accepted as an unfortunate, yet normal, side effect of the time of the month. However, Chinese medical texts tell us something different:

'It is not normal to have pain; pain shows dysfunction.'[1]
The nature of menstrual pain can help to diagnose what might be wrong:

- Pain where a hot water bottle is needed to soothe – Cold
- Pain accompanied by a fever – Heat
- Generalized aching pain – Qi Stagnation
- Localized stabbing pain – Blood Stagnation

Other menstrual-related symptoms

Spotting or bleeding

Spotting before a period:

- if the blood is bright red – Heat, or
- if the spotting is brownish – weak Qi or Blood (requires rest and moxibustion).
- Spotting after menstruation – Qi Stagnation or Blood Stagnation.
- Spotting after ovulation indicates a deficiency in the luteal phase (the latter phase of the menstrual cycle, or post-ovulation phase) – this can be caused by a number of reasons including low progesterone levels. See Chapter Six for more on ovulation.

Note: spotting about eight days after ovulation can also be a sign of implantation (see page 218).

Pain around ovulation

This is not considered normal, but can be a sign of ovulation. If it is followed by scant or sparse bleeding it can indicate Yin Deficiency (see page 129).

Cervical mucus

You may notice increased vaginal secretions mid-cycle. This cervical or 'fertile' mucus is produced to help the passage of the sperm. Ideally, it needs to be like egg whites – clear and slippery in texture. Check it by stretching it between your fingers – you should be able to stretch it into a long strand between your thumb and forefinger. Healthy, clear cervical mucus is a sign that you are about to ovulate and that you are fertile.

If your mucus is not clear and like egg whites, then this could indicate low fertility. If your mucus is thick and yellow this could indicate Damp/Heat. If it is thick and white, this could indicate Damp/Cold, and if it is scanty or absent this can indicate Blood Deficient or Heat.

If you are experiencing an unpleasant odour, redness, swelling or itching, or highly discoloured discharge, you may have an infection and need to see the GP.

Premenstrual symptoms that indicate Qi Stagnation:
- Swollen abdomen
- Water retention
- Tender and swollen breasts
- Moodiness and irritability; being prone to angry outbursts
- Loose stools or constipation

Some of my patients report significant premenstrual symptoms from mid-cycle (ovulation) for two weeks until their period arrives. This is usually an indication of severe Qi Stagnation.

In my experience, the body's response to treatment is often seen first in the menstrual symptoms. The pain may ease, the blood may be different, the cycle regulates; these are often positive and encouraging indicators for patients, showing that the treatment is having an effect.

Q&A

I have had an irregular menstrual cycle since my periods started and I was on the Pill for ten years. Will this make it harder to treat me?
Everyone responds differently, I have had patients who have never had regular cycles regulate within a couple of menstrual cycles but there are those who take longer. Nearly everyone who follows my baby-making plan will see some improvements fairly quickly. It is true that if the problem has been around for a long time then it will take longer to fix. However, I advise my patients to *choose* for it to change quickly. There is evidence to suggest if we believe something is going to be hard to treat – it will be; so stay positive.

Your general appearance

In Chinese medicine, a patient's appearance – from their hair to the way they walk and talk – can reveal a lot about their overall vitality and health.

In the clinic, I consider several factors to obtain a deeper analysis of the emotional and physical wellbeing of my patients.

The eyes

The eyes are important for diagnosis in both Western and Chinese medicine, and are often referred to as a 'window to the soul'. They give information on the health of the liver and on emotions, both of which are key players in fertility. Eyes betray tiredness, a night out, sadness, hurt and – at the other end of the spectrum – joy and glee.

CASE STUDY: HOT-BLOODED

A case I found particularly interesting was that of a patient who had a great deal of Heat in her body: her tongue was red, she was restless and agitated and suffered from night sweats. I treated her weekly for three weeks before her period. When it arrived, it was a great deal heavier than usual and bright red. She also woke up in the night with a nosebleed – again the blood was bright red.

After this, her entire system cooled down; she was a great deal calmer and no longer had night sweats. I had given her acupuncture to rid the body of Heat

and it's possible that her heavy period and the nosebleed were the means by which the body could do that. She didn't have another nosebleed and her periods after that were not as heavy or bright red.

The role of acupuncture in Chinese medicine is to enable the body to function at its best. The success of acupuncture depends on how severe the symptoms are, as well as the quality of a patient's Qi, Jing and Shen. This case demonstrates how big changes can take place with simple techniques and minimal intervention.

Western doctors can tell from a yellowing of the eyes, if a patient has jaundice. It is a sign of severe liver disease, or even that the liver has packed up completely. A light yellow tinge to the sclera (white of the eye) can also indicate that someone is regularly over-indulging; their liver is overworked, having to break down and process alcohol.

Ideally we would like our eyes to be clear, to 'sparkle' (whereby the light catches and bounces off them) and to have vitality. Take a mirror and see if your eyes fit one of the descriptions below:

- **Cloudy** – this can indicate an unsettled mind and Qi Stagnation.
- **Dull** – this can indicate an emotional issue that needs to be addressed.
- **Red** – this can indicate Heat and tiredness (Blood Deficient).
- **Yellowing in the whites of the eyes** – shows ill health and Qi deficiency.
- **Puffy** – this can be caused by Dampness.
- **Dark rings** – a well-recognized sign that you are not getting enough sleep. It can also signify reproductive weakness.
- **Weeping or watery** – you may literally be grieving or sad and showing tears you are unable to cry.
- **Red, weeping and watery** – this can be hay fever, which is sometimes a symptom of Damp.
- **Bloodshot** – this can indicate suppressed anger.

Eyes and emotions

Clear eyes in Chinese medicine, denote someone's ability not only to 'see' in the literal sense, but also to 'have vision', in terms of their direction in life and their ability to plan ahead. The idea of vision is very important in fertility because children are bound up with the idea of the future.

The frustration suffered by patients who have tried for a long time to conceive is often visible in their eyes. They are unable to plan ahead and their energy 'stagnates'. Many patients with fertility issues suffer from Qi Stagnation (see page 132).

I think it's no coincidence that visualization has proved so helpful to those trying to enhance the natural function of the Liver in Chinese medicine. The act of visualizing our desires and focusing on our long-term goals is healthy for the Liver and for the movement of the Liver Qi.

EYE TREATMENTS

For itchy eyes Try either nettle tea or 'palming' – rub your palms together vigorously until they generate heat, then cup your hands over your eyes for a minute. You can do this as often as you like.

For dry, red eyes Try an eye mask that you can make at home: slice a cold cucumber very thinly and put into a damp muslin cloth. Store in the fridge for a while, then lie down and place over your eyes. This is actually soothing and moisturizing. If the cloth is very slightly damp it will hold the slices in place next to your skin while your relax.

Alternatively, try chrysanthemum tea. Pour boiling water on to the dried chrysanthemum flower heads – which you can buy from good health food or Chinese medicine shops. Leave to brew for a few minutes and strain. Drink some of the tea – it's good for the eyes and also aids digestion – and leave some to cool. Then, dampen a flat cotton pad in the cooled, strained tea and use to bathe your eyes.

A good eye exercise for tired and sore eyes is to imagine the eye as the face of a clock; start by directing your gaze at twelve on your imaginary clock, then move your eyes – using just the eye muscles, not your whole head – to one, then two, then three and so on, until you have gone full circle.

Eyes and the spirit

As well as revealing a lot about your health, the eyes can also give away something of your 'spirit' (or Shen; see page 88). Those with a strong spirit often respond well to first-line treatments such as acupuncture and changes to diet. If the spirit recovers and is strong, the prognosis is good. Those whose spirit has been weakened or is 'ungrounded' (as is often the case with those who regularly use drugs), however, often need deeper emotional work and sometimes support from professionals in other fields.

The mouth and lips

Chinese medicine makes a connection between the health of our digestive system and the appearance of our mouth and lips. Problems here can reveal digestive disturbance and the secrets of how we are nourishing ourselves. And factors such as swollen lips, for example, can be indicative of both health and emotional issues.

The colour of lips

The normal colour and condition of lips is pale red, moist and slightly shiny. However, they can also be:

- **pale with a bluish or purple tinge** – Cold
- **very red** – Heat
- **pale and dry** – Blood Deficient
- **cracked at the corners** – this can indicate a Vitamin B deficiency and a supplement such as folic acid which is key for conception and pregnancy should be taken
- **greenish in hue** – Qi Stagnation
- **swollen** – indicating problems with the digestive system; Damp

In addition, if you suffer from cold sores, this can point to localized Damp Heat, while spots on the chin may indicate Blood Stagnation.

The tongue

Your tongue gives up a great deal of information about your health and is, perhaps, one of the most famous diagnostic tools in Chinese medicine.

Of course, practitioners use more than just a tongue chart. In my study at home, I have thudding great books that chart even minuscule differences in the condition of the tongue. I'm not going to go into that level of detail here, and have boiled it down into broad categories

Colour, coat and texture

The ideal tongue colour is pale red. It should be slightly wet, with no significant marks. Colour variations may include:

- **red** – Heat
- **purple** – Stagnation
- **pale** – Blood Deficiency
- **orange sides** – Blood Deficiency
- **red tip** – Heat in the heart (indicating anxiety; often these patients have disturbed sleep)
- **blue** – Cold/Blood Stagnation.

As for coat/texture, a tongue that is:

- heavily coated is a sign of poor digestive function and Dampness; the patient will usually be a little sluggish and may feel general malaise
- dirty brown or thick and yellow in colour can indicate Damp Heat
- white and thick shows a tendency towards Cold/Damp
- cracked along the centre can point to poor digestion, but is generally indicative of Yin Deficiency or Heat
- veined underneath can tell us a lot about the condition of the Blood.

In addition, teeth marks can indicate poor digestive function (the tongue is swollen, hence you get teeth marks), while a tongue that quivers involuntarily indicates Qi Deficiency.

Like the pulse, the tongue is an excellent tool for monitoring changes in a patient's health. It also has the advantage of being much easier to read.

My patients sometimes hesitate before sticking their tongues out for fear of what I will read, particularly male patients. Recently, a male patient widened his eyes when I asked to see his tongue, then launched into a quick confession: 'Look, you'll know anyway, but I was out for a curry and beers with the boys last night – please don't tell my wife; I told her I wasn't drinking!'

On another occasion, I was alarmed when I saw the tongue of a patient who had recently miscarried. I saw strong evidence of severe Blood Stagnation and suspected that the miscarriage had been incomplete. I immediately started writing out a referral for her to a gynaecologist, when she confirmed my suspicions: 'I have to have an operation tomorrow,' she said. 'I had a scan yesterday that showed that I have what they call "retained products of conception".'

Skin

Skin, the largest organ of the human body, reveals a lot about a person's health. I often tell patients that by looking at the condi-

---

DRY SKIN BRUSHING

Very useful to get the Qi moving around the body, the skin is the largest organ of the body, and by stimulating it through brushing you are encouraging the natural elimination function. Damp types and Stagnant types really benefit from this, but it is suitable for all.

I also recommend it for patients in between IVF to help the lymphatic system in preparation for the IVF drugs. Brush before a shower or bath, once or twice a day.

- Use a long-handled, natural-fibred bristle brush
- Always brush towards the heart
- Start with the soles of the feet
- Brush up the legs towards the torso
- Brush from the tips of the fingers to the shoulders
- Brush over the buttocks
- Use light pressure only on the stomach if you think you might be pregnant. Trace the direction of the intestines from right to left
- Enjoy the tingling feeling of the Qi moving around the body and follow with a warm bath or shower

tion of their skin, I am doing the Chinese medicine version of reading their medical records. For the purpose of this diagnosis, I am going to talk about the overall colour and condition of the skin (body and face):

- **Redness** – Heat
- **A very oily complexion** – Damp
- **Weeping sores** – Damp Heat
- **Itchy skin** – Blood Deficient
- **Noticeable pallor** – often means Blood Deficient
- **Dry skin** – Blood Deficient
- **Puffy skin that leaves an indent** – Dampness and fluid retention
- **Breakouts on the chin** – can indicate Stagnation and/or Damp Heat in the reproductive system.

EMOTIONS AND DIET

A common mistake made by both patients and practitioners is thinking they can compensate in one area by overcompensating in another. This is particularly true of the diet. Food can, of course, affect both the engine and the mind, and there is a great deal of evidence to show that by improving diet, mood and behaviour can be altered. However, I would suggest that it is better to direct the treatment to where the problem lies and that requires good diagnostic skills. If the diet is central to the problem, then changing it will have far-reaching consequences; but if it's the mind that is central to the problem, changing the diet will not achieve much in the long term.

Many patients who are struggling with the mind use diet as a way of controlling their emotions – so giving them more dietary advice only feeds into their need to control things in this way. I find that with these patients, the more out of control they are the more controlling they become. So by changing their diet radically they may well *feel* like they are back in control but are they really?

Does your skin have another 'tinge' to it?
- **Yellow** – suggests problems with the liver
- **Green** – Stagnation
- **Black** – localized congestion, Blood Stagnation

Do you sweat?
Excessive sweating can be indicative of Heat (especially if you are throwing off the covers at night), Yin Deficiency (an advanced state of Heat) or Dampness.

Hair

I look at the quality and condition of the hair. In Chinese medicine hair quality reflects the quality of the blood.

I am always concerned about a woman's hormonal health when she reports suffering hair loss. If this applies to you, I suggest that you follow the cycle for a Blood Deficient type (see page 121) and really moderate your exercise. Chicken soup is great for blood nourishment (see page 50), along with a good book and an early night!

Your system

Your urine

The colour, amount and frequency of urine are also assessed. A healthy, well-hydrated person passes between 1 and 2 litres of urine a day, which means they go to the loo around five to seven times. Ideally, your urine should be clear, but very slightly yellow. However, it may be:
- **cloudy** – Dampness
- **very frequent** – weak Qi
- **plentiful and clear** – Cold
- **dark and scanty** – Heat (and dehydration)
  Dribbling after urination indicates weak Qi.

Your stools

Yes, I'm sorry, your stools (that is, your poo) are also scrutinized in Chinese medicine. Ideally, we would all pass perfectly formed stools shortly after rising in the morning. However, as most people tumble out of bed, then hit the ground running, a perfectly formed stool is not on their list of priorities.

In clinic, I do ask my patients how often they have a bowel movement. The answers are really very varied. Some patients do go every day, but others go an entire week without one. These are all possibilities:

- **Constipation, followed by small, bitty stools** ('rabbit droppings') – Qi Stagnation
- **Constipation with pain and a cold tummy** – Cold or Damp/Cold
- **Constipation where the stool is dry** – Blood Deficient or Heat
- **Constipation followed by diarrhoea** (typical of irritable bowel syndrome) – Qi Stagnation
- **Strong-smelling stools** – Damp/Heat
- **Mucus in stools** – Damp
- **Black or dark stools** – Blood Stagnation
- **Wind** – normally indicates Qi Stagnation
- **Wind with strong smell** – Damp/Heat

Sleep

Sleep is very important (see pages 36–41). Sleep problems are very often linked with Blood Deficiency. In Chinese medicine, it's said: 'If the Blood is not strong, then the mind cannot settle and the sleep is disturbed.' I can tell if a patient is having dream-disturbed sleep or if they are anxious because the very tip of their tongue will be red.

My father used to say: 'Big brain – small sleep; small brain

– big sleep.' He was plagued by insomnia his entire life, mostly because he suffered from tinnitus, but also because he had so many thoughts rattling around in his head. There are lots of points on the sole of the foot that help you sleep so I suggest you – or your partner – massage your feet an hour before bedtime if you are having problems sleeping. I often massage my daughters' feet before bed if they are frightened or have problems sleeping. Here are some tips to help you sleep:

- Don't eat late in the evening.
- Steer clear of anything that might be stimulating, such as coffee, after supper.
- Eat light at night – a heavy meal may 'sit' in your stomach.
- Avoid serious discussions before bed.
- Don't work before bed.

How emotions impact on health

Emotional wellbeing is a particularly interesting area in fertility, especially when you have a case of what Western medicine terms, 'unexplained infertility'. In Chinese medicine, intense or difficult emotions are considered to be a cause of physical problems and even disease. Increasingly, I am finding that I do a lot of work in this area in my clinic.

Rebalancing your emotions may play a large part in your fertility journey; Chinese medicine sees a direct connection between the Heart and the Womb (there is a lovely yoga exercise in the Appendix that concentrates on reconnecting the two – see page 349).

Some patients have experienced an obvious trauma, but may not have fully realized the impact that this has had on their life and health. It's certainly the case that, in an effort to get on, many people underplay issues in their lives that bother them – even if they have upset them quite fundamentally. You may even find, when you think about it, that your chief symptom first appeared during a period of emotional uncertainty.

However, emotional stress does not have to come from acute trauma. It can also evolve from low-grade and consistent exposure to difficult emotional situations – a difficult or bullying boss, caring for a sick relative or medical problems, for example. These can have a 'wearing-down' effect.

You should, by now, have compiled a comprehensive list of symptoms and areas that are concerning you. Perhaps you have identified some Cold symptoms or Qi Deficiency? Or you may be able to see where your health might be out of

MEN – WHAT CAN YOU DO?

Be supportive. Accompany your partner on her journey, hold her hand, ask her how she feels and ask her about what she is learning. The presence, and by that I mean emotional *and* physical presence, of the male partner on this journey towards a healthy conception can make a big difference to the outcome.

A couple of years ago, I did an audit of my patients. I compared the time taken by women who attended my clinic with their partners to get pregnant, with the time it took those women who came alone. There were 32 per cent more pregnancies over a six-

month period in the group where both partners came for treatment.

There are two obvious reasons for this. Firstly, the men in the first group made a conscious effort to get on board and to improve the quality of their sperm. I always offer men the chance to get involved, and I will even recommend another practitioner if they prefer not to share. But secondly, I am also certain that the support a woman *feels* when her partner is involved is invaluable to the process of conception and that too makes for a positive outcome.

There is a 'male cycle' on page 196 – look at it and join in!

balance and how you can start to implement small lifestyle changes. This is whole-body health, and with a little work, you can create that fertile soil I talked about at the beginning of the chapter. Remember, each change that you make for the better can have far-reaching effects on your health and fertility and bring you a step closer to that longed-for pregnancy.

In Chapter Three you are going to move on to looking at more detail at your fertility type and specific recommendations for each type. You will get more specific advice on how to create balance and optimize each phase of your menstrual cycle in Part Two (Chapters Four to Seven).

Chapter Three

Your fertility type

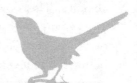

W hen I sat down to write this book, my aim was to give my readers – you – some simple tools to work with. I wanted to provide you with something empowering that would put you in the driving seat and allow you to take control of your own fertility. And I wanted the process to be fun and enjoyable.

With this in mind, I decided that being able to determine your fertility type or tendencies would, in turn, put you in a position to follow a comprehensive plan to rebalance your system and get fit for conception.

We touched on some symptoms in the last two chapters, and now we're going to tackle each type head on, so that you can really see which description best fits your current state. To do this, read the descriptions below and find the statements and symptoms you most closely identify with.

And remember, if you show a tendency towards a particular fertility type, it does not mean you are stuck with that label for ever. The aim here is to rebalance you away from that tendency and restore you to a centred and balanced 'ideal' state – the place you want to be at the moment you conceive your baby.

Your type may also change over time. In my life, for example, I have had symptoms of Heat in my system (when I was on very strong medical treatment) and I have also been Blood Deficient (after giving birth to my children). The idea is to balance symptoms gently, whenever you see them arise.

As already mentioned, most people are strong candidates for more than one type, and if that is the case with you, you should follow the recommendations for both types so that you can rebalance both. As you read the descriptions, you will also get an idea from how closely you identify with them, how long you have been in a given condition. If you feel that you've had certain tendencies for a long time, I'd advise you to repeat the cycles in Part Two at least four times. Follow the advice for your type with each cycle. Stick with it and don't be put off. It may take some concentrated effort to rid yourself of, say, a Damp condition, but it will be worth it. You will feel better than you have ever felt before. And you will be in the perfect zone to prepare for conception. Remember to keep it simple and go with the main symptom.

Again, jot down all your ideas on a piece of paper, so that you can build a comprehensive picture of all the areas you could address. Once you have completed this chapter, you will start your treatment and set out on the exciting journey ahead to conception. Keep that image of your healthy pregnancy in mind – let's not forget why we are doing this!

What part do you play in all of this?

You play the biggest part. Learning and understanding what tendencies you have, and then effecting the necessary changes to bring about good, balanced health, puts you right in the driving seat of this programme. It helps you to understand your health and your physical and emotional needs, then act accordingly.

I do, occasionally, see patients who simply go through the motions and do not *engage* in the process. This approach will not change your life, and all I can do in such cases is damage limitation.

How quickly will you see an improvement?

As I have explained, this depends on how entrenched the condition has become. If a problem started early in life and you are now thirty-three, it may take some months to see an improvement. That said, I also see patients who improve immediately, then plateau for a bit before improving again. Sometimes patients see very little improvement for some time and then experience a rapid recovery.

In general, you should expect to see gradual improvements over a period of a few cycles with highs and lows along the way. I do also think it is important not to rule out the occasional miracle – we do certainly see them in the clinic, when even the most stubborn cases sometimes miraculously

KEEPING IT SIMPLE

Humans lead increasingly complicated lives and tend to overcomplicate their *approach* to life too. This can be seen in the plethora of fertility treatments and medicines that is available, and in the way that people often reach for them before even trying the simple approach, which sometimes does the job best.

Anyone who is thinking of fertility medicine should try this simple approach first. It cannot harm to be in peak health, and it is an enjoyable and, above all, empowering plan too. As I often say to my patients: 'Make life changes with joy in your heart.'

turn around. I have seen spontaneous healing with my own eyes, and it's worth bearing in mind that pregnancies can be achieved in the most unlikely situations. There's a big sign in my clinic that says, 'Expect a miracle'. Which means, don't give up on yourself.

How do you become a specific type?

The Chinese believe that we are all born with a tendency towards one type or another. However, conditions sometimes develop as a result of lifestyle and living conditions. For example, someone may be Blood Deficient through years of overwork, heavy periods from a young age and an irregular diet. Or they may suddenly become Blood Deficient following an acute episode of blood loss through, say, miscarriage, birth or an accident. We'll look at all this in more detail below.

What happens if you have two types and their treatment is contradictory?

Occasionally, this can make treatment difficult, for example if you are both a Damp and a Blood Deficient person – the treatment for Damp requires that you get moving, but if you are Blood Deficient you need to rest.

Despite this, it is possible to incorporate both into a plan because I have adapted the treatment around the menstrual cycle, and different conditions have more (or less) significance at different times of the cycles. The post-period phase is not a good time for Blood Deficient types for obvious reasons, but there is relief for those with Heat in their system, even if they suffer a heavy bleed. The effects of Damp are more significant during ovulation, when the egg is released and there is more fluid around. A Damp and Blood Deficient patient needs, therefore, to relax and rest during her period – an important time for this type – and get out and about and moving during ovulation, when it is important to compensate for the slowing effect of having Damp in the system. So, let's get down to business. Once again, I am going to look at the following broad categories:

- Cold
- Damp
- Blood Deficient
- Heat
- Stagnant (separated into Liver Qi and Blood)

Are you Cold?

About 20–30 per cent of patients I see in my fertility clinic have a tendency to Cold, and occasionally I see a patient who is acutely Cold (see the case study on page 116). If you are Cold, you will probably find yourself agreeing with between five and eight of the statements below:

- You have an abdomen that is cold to touch.
- You have water retention (i.e. puffiness on the body, especially the abdomen and legs).
- You go to the loo frequently, and produce a lot of clear urine.
- You have loose bowel movements.
- You take longer to finish things – you're a 'slow burner'.
- It takes you a while to build up enthusiasm.
- You have a white coat on your tongue.
- You are pale – even slightly blueish on occasion.
- You have a sluggish digestion.
- You put on weight easily.
- You have a medium to low libido (sexual appetite).
- You would rather stay in with a good book, a cuddle and a hot-water bottle.

- You feel worse in cold weather.
- You would rather take a holiday on the beach than go skiing.
- You sleep deeply.
- You find you often sit near or on the radiator.

How does Cold affect your fertility?

A Cold condition can mean that the flow of blood to the uterus is inhibited because the blood vessels are contracted. This means that Cold types often suffer from periods that are late, painful (perhaps where a hot-water bottle is needed to soothe) or scanty.

What makes you Cold?

Some people have a natural tendency towards Cold, and then environmental factors exacerbate their condition. Common environmental factors are:

- eating too much cold food
- eating raw food
- drinking cold water – where possible drink water at room temperature
- drinking or eating food directly from the fridge
- spending too much time in cold rooms – whether because they are under-heated or over-air-conditioned
- certain prescription and over-the-counter drugs, including anaesthetics, antibiotics, antidiuretics, antacids and tranquillizers – these can either make a Cold type worse or even push someone into a Cold condition.

When I am working through a patient's fertility type, I will often ask them to describe how they feel at home and at the office. If you are exposed to too much external cold, you may find you are increasingly a Cold type. When you are cold the body has to work hard to warm up; this weakens it and can cause physical complaints, among them issues with fertility. These are the kinds of environmental questions you may need to answer:

- How many outside walls are there in your bedroom?
- Where is your bed, is it near the window?
- Is your home draughty?
- Do you walk on cold floors with bare feet?
- Do you sit on cold surfaces?
- Is there air conditioning in your office; if so, is your desk near the unit?
- Are you sitting still for long periods of time?

Immediate steps to help deal with Cold tendencies

Do:
- drink teas, such as ginger tea
- eat 'warming' foods (as described in full on page 161)
- eat predominantly cooked food, including cooked or stewed fruit
- add ginger to my basic chicken soup recipe (see page 50)
- stay cosy – if necessary with blankets
- take warming baths with essential oils such as bergamot, orange, cardamom, cinnamon
- sleep away from the window and from any draughts (such as air vents)
- practise yoga stretches
- try vigorous breathing techniques such as panting (but not hyperventilating!).

Don't:
- eat food straight the fridge
- drink cold liquids
- eat raw food.

CASE STUDY: TWO COLD CASES

CASE STUDY ONE

Cold case one is about Sally, a thirty-four-year-old executive who had been Cold for a long time, but environmental factors were exacerbating her condition. She travelled a lot on long-haul over-air-conditioned flights, and when she first arrived in my clinic I noted that she was slightly overweight with lack of 'form' (her skin was soft and doughy to the touch) and moved slowly, as if she lacked energy.

In the course of our consultation, she described how she found it difficult to lose weight and felt she had eaten 'a lifetime's supply' of salad to absolutely no effect. She made fruit smoothies for breakfast, taking the ingredients directly from the fridge and blending them fresh to avoid losing the valuable vitamins.

She said that her menstrual cycles were long and sometimes painful and, in an attempt to deal with this, she took a lot of painkillers, particularly Nurofen Plus, and used a hot-water bottle over her tummy.

Later, she mentioned that she always felt cold at home; there were two outside walls in her bedroom, and her side of the bed was by the window. She added that she often argued with her husband about whether to sleep with the window open or closed.

Sally was clearly long-term Cold. She'd been trying to conceive for three years – two of those years with effort.

I suggested immediately that the bed should be moved so that it was next to a warm wall and that Sally should switch sides with her partner so that she was not sleeping near the window or any draught.

To her relief, I took her off her self-imposed salad 'starvation' and suggested instead warm, nourishing foods, such as chicken soup with added ginger. I added garlic, cardamom, cinnamon, rosemary, root vegetables and lentils to her diet (see chapters four to seven for more information on which foods are recommended for which type) and sent her away with a recipe for slow-roasted root vegetables with rosemary and garlic for her supper. I also asked her to replace her morning smoothie with a ginger tea and try some stewed apples with cinnamon in her porridge. She was forbidden to eat ice cream.

Sally was reluctant to give up the painkillers, as she had relied on them for so long, but I persuaded her to try some yoga exercises to help manage her period pain. I also suggested that she should rest more at that time of her cycle, taking warm baths and getting early nights. Finally, I recommended she travelled long haul with her own warm, non-static blanket (she disliked those provided by the airlines).

continued overleaf...

CASE STUDY: TWO COLD CASES *continued...*

It took four months for Sally to warm up, but she did. She saw an immediate improvement in her menstrual cycle, but it took a little longer for everything else to fall into balance. This is common in Chinese medicine and it's called 'flight to health': a massive difference, followed by a slow climb with occasional setbacks.

She went through four cycles, but I put in a lot of additions for someone who was Cold, with particular emphasis on the post-menstrual phase.

CASE STUDY TWO
Cold case two describes a woman becoming acutely cold over forty-eight hours. Victoria, who happens to be a friend as well as a patient, came to the clinic having just driven back from France. She had been on the road for two days in mid-summer and the air conditioning

had been unintentionally trained on her stomach for the entire trip.

She arrived in my clinic shortly afterwards and her abdomen was still freezing cold to the touch. She said her stools were loose, and I noticed a blue hue around her lips. I gave her acupuncture with moxibustion as a first-line treatment. Then I sent her home with instructions for how to do an abdominal massage, vigorous breathing techniques (panting) and yoga stretches. I suggested some warming essential oils (such as bergamot, orange, cardamom, cinnamon) and instructed her to add a lot of ginger to her chicken soup. I forbade her from eating anything straight from the fridge or anything raw.

Although acute when she arrived, Victoria's symptoms were very quick to respond to treatment.

Are you Damp?

Damp is the term used to describe an overly moist or wet condition, where fluids have accumulated inappropriately. This is what happens when fluids become too thick and viscous to permeate the membranes of the body. Damp has a sluggish, stagnant, stuck quality. It is heavy and sticky and can be obstructive. Phlegm is the more congealed form of Dampness.

In Chinese medicine having polycystic ovarian syndrome (PCOS) often falls into the category of excess Damp condition. Water retention, bloating, excess weight, fatigue, lack of appetite, a heavy feeling in the body or limbs, heavy head, cysts, yeasts, excess mucus, Candida, allergies, thrush, eczema, asthma, arthritis, tumours, excess weight, cellulite, watery or loose stools, weakness and feeling cold and/or lethargic are all indicators of an excess Damp condition.

The corresponding emotions that a Damp condition engenders are worry and anxiety. When your internal communication is hindered or inhibited, this gives rise to the feeling of worry, which strongly inhibits the digestion, then exaccrbates the Damp condition, creating a negative mind–body loop.

I think it's no coincidence that the number of cases of Damp in the UK, is on the increase – our weather doesn't help, for a start. I imagine my Californian colleagues see far fewer in their dry climate. Around half of the patients I see have symptoms of Dampness – it may be immediately obvious, as in cases of Candida and allergies, or it may be well hidden, as with some mild forms of polycystic ovaries. If you have already been diagnosed with polycystic ovaries, you need to read this section, and follow the recommendations for Damp.

It's worth noting that I often see patients with both Damp and Heat, so if you recognize something of yourself here, you should take a look at the Heat section too. And Damp can also be seen with Cold.

Dampness is a tricky one to treat – it takes dedication both on the part of the practitioner and the patient. But stick with it. The results can be amazing, particularly if you have been struggling with weight issues. If you agree with between five and eight of the following statements, you may have features of Damp:

- You suffer from allergies, such as asthma or hay fever.
- You suffer from skin conditions that appear 'wet', e.g. eczema.

- You have an oily complexion.
- You suffer from Candida or thrush.
- You have thick cervical mucus.
- There is mucus in your stools.
- You experience fungal infections of the skin.
- Your build is very slim, yet you have cellulite.
- You prefer a sedentary life.
- You 'crash' when you fall asleep.
- Your legs feel heavy.
- You have a lot of cellulite.[1]
- You feel bloated for a long time after you eat, and your food 'sits' in your stomach.
- You feel 'stuck' in life?
- You find it difficult to concentrate.
- You have a fuzzy head. (Dampness is said to 'mist the mind'.)
- You experience foul-smelling stools. (See also Heat, below.)

How does Damp affect your fertility?

As I said, Damp is a stubborn one, and if you think you have Damp symptoms, get on with making the changes I recommend as soon as you can.

In terms of the menstrual cycle, Damp can affect the passage of the egg through the Fallopian tube, slowing it down or even causing it to be obstructed. This means the egg can miss its window for implantation. It may also coat the womb lining in a thick layer making it difficult for the egg to implant successfully. Damp may also clog the ovaries so that they are unable to release an egg, as in PCOS.

What makes you Damp?

Common contributing factors to being Damp include:
- a diet that's too rich in heavy, fatty foods

CASE STUDY: CLEARING DAMP

It is sometimes possible to see the damp release while treating a Damp patient. I once had a pregnant patient with acute Dampness, which had manifested as oedema in her ankles. As I was treating her with acupuncture the fluid started leaving her body, and afterwards she was visibly less oedemic. When she swung her legs around to get off the treatment bed, I noticed that she'd left two holes in the paper where it had become so wet it had torn under her heels.

- STDs – these are often classified as Damp Heat, so if you have suffered from an STD in the past it often leaves a legacy of Damp in the system, such as Chlamydia; patients with this silent but damaging disease can have blocked Fallopian tubes
- birth-control pills (the contraceptive pill) and the morning-after pill
- antibiotics
- some of the drugs used in IVF, including steroids
- living in a basement
- exposure to a damp environment
- alcohol – particularly beer
- dairy products – vegetarians who eat a lot of dairy foods can have Damp symptoms
- too many processed foods
- too much sugar
- a sedentary lifestyle
- overeating.

Note: Dampness can also cause Blood Deficiency in the long term because it inhibits the digestive system and thus the body's ability to 'make' blood, so if you have identified Damp symptoms in yourself, please check the entry on Blood Deficiency as well (see page 121).

Immediate steps to help deal with Damp tendencies

I'm sorry to say that the diet for clearing Damp is unbelievably dull. But the good news is that you will feel better quickly and, in the longer term, you will feel lighter and more 'alive'. I strongly recommend that you cut out or avoid:

- alcohol (especially beer)
- dairy foods (especially cheese)
- chocolate
- curries (especially if you are Damp/Heat)
- bread
- wheat in other forms, such as cakes, biscuits, etc.
- fried foods
- sugar
- ready-cracked nuts (these are Damp-forming because the oil is exposed to the air), including peanuts, walnuts, almonds, pistachios, cashews.

In addition to the above, **don't**:

- drink too much water[2]
- eat too late at night (most people are usually inactive after eating and this can lead to Damp accumulation)
- eat proteins and carbohydrates together – complicated meals with lots of different food groups can further aggravate the problem, but meat and salad would be fine, as would pasta and vegetables; you could also try the Hay Diet (see Resources).

Even if you can only manage a temporary hiatus, I really need you to break the cycle with these foods. You then need to lighten your diet considerably. I recommend that you include:

- fresh foods
- lots of bitter leaves (e.g. frisée and watercress)

- barley water (see recipe, below)
- onions
- garlic
- aduki beans or any small red bean
- alfalfa sprouts
- celery
- chicory
- fennel
- jasmine tea, green tea, fennel tea
- herbs and spices, such as cardamom, ginger, sage, thyme, parsley.

Are you Blood Deficient?

Many women are Blood Deficient, and perhaps as many as 60 per cent of the women I see have an element of Blood Deficiency. It does not necessarily mean that you are anaemic, but it may mean that you are on the road to iron-deficiency anaemia.

In Chinese medicine, Blood is 'made' from the food we eat. The key to getting back to health for a Blood Deficient type is, simply put, to get good, regular nutrition, adequate rest and introduce structured working times, so that there is no danger of overwork. I also seriously recommend that they reduce or cut out alcohol. Those with Blood Deficiency should complete at least four of my cycles to ensure that they are completely back on track.

Blood Deficiency can manifest in one of two ways – either physically or emotionally.

Barley Water

150g of pearl barley

1 tbsp finely grated ginger (only for Cold types) – boil with the barley

2 lemons: grate the zest and then juice them, setting aside the liquid

4 tablespoons of honey

1.5 litres of water

Rinse the barley under a tap, until the water runs clear, and put in a saucepan. Add the lemon zest, and ginger (if using). Bring the mixture to the boil and then simmer for ten minutes. Strain the liquid into a cooking bowl and throw away the used barley. Stir in the honey a tablespoon at a time allowing it to dissolve in the mixture. Finally, pour in the lemon juice and stir before setting the mixture to one side to cool. Decant into bottles. Damp types can store this in the fridge but I recommend that you drink it at room temperature.

121

Physical symptoms can be tiredness, eye ticks, itching, general dryness of the skin and hair, whereas emotional symptoms are more likely to present as anxieties and problems sleeping.

Unlike Damp types, those with a Blood Deficient condition have an attractive road to recovery. It's about indulging yourself – being kind to yourself, rather than following a rigorous dietary regime. However, you also need to learn to say 'No', and to know when to stop. This is often a challenge.

You may be Blood Deficient if you agree with five to eight of the following statements:

CASE STUDY: BLOOD DEFICIENT

Very recently, I had a patient who had 'recovered' from a bout of malaria. When I say recovered, she had finished her course of medication and had been told by the hospital that all her parasites had been cleared.

She threw herself straight back into work and life resumed as normal. She went out in the evening, she had the odd glass of wine and she ran around spinning those metaphorical plates simultaneously.

However, after one week she was almost bent double with exhaustion, she was seeing black 'floaters' in front of her eyes and she was so tired by the end of the day she was unable to move – literally. She went to her GP who was very worried about her condition and referred her back to the hospital to make sure that the parasites had not returned.

She was again given the all-clear, but told me she had been 'shattered' for four weeks, was unable to go out and had gone 'completely off' alcohol. She looked like a ghost, but was not technically anaemic (her blood had been checked by the hospital).

I immediately identified her as severely Blood Deficient with physical symptoms. Her hair was dry, she had broken nails and she felt 'itchy'.

I treated her with acupuncture and put her on a diet of greens, greens and more greens, lentils and red meat. I also insisted she see a herbalist. I told her she must rest as a matter of urgency and hibernate until she felt steadier on her feet.

Her recovery will take at least four cycles, but she is committed and has already improved.

- You have a scant menstrual flow or amenorrhoea (no periods at all).
- You have a pale complexion.
- You have dull, dry skin.
- You have dry hair.
- Your lips and tongue are pale.
- Your nails are dry and brittle.
- There is an orange tinge on the sides of your tongue.
- You experience dizziness.
- You see spots in front of your eyes (called floaters).
- You are often forgetful or scatty.
- Your colleagues describe you as a workaholic.
- You find it difficult to fall asleep.
- You feel unsettled when you lie in bed.
- You experience feelings of anxiety and sometimes feel a rising panic in your chest.
- You are prone to panic attacks.
- Your mind is restless – lack of concentration.
- You are easily startled.
- You have a slim build.
- You catch everything that's going around.
- You are the last to leave work.

How does Blood Deficiency affect your fertility?

Although some Blood Deficient patients have had heavy periods at some point in their lives, by the time they present to me, they have scant periods or, sometimes, none at all. The period is obviously an essential phase of the menstrual cycle.

Blood Deficient types tend to have problems generating enough blood to thicken the endometrium (womb lining) sufficiently, so that it is not thick enough to be able to maintain a pregnancy. The womb lining needs to be 8mm thick at implantation.

What makes you Blood Deficient?

Many things can cause Blood Deficiency, not least a straight-forward loss of blood, such as a miscarriage or after child-birth. In Chinese medicine we say that one drop of mother's milk takes one drop of mother's Blood, which means that mothers who breastfeed for longer than six months may find themselves Blood Deficient and need to nourish their Blood while continuing to feed their baby.

Environmental contributors can be a sudden shock – such as a car accident. (A miscarriage gives you a double whammy because it is both shocking and involves actual blood loss.) Illnesses can also be a root cause, particularly if you haven't tak-en enough time off to recover. These include viruses, bacterial illnesses or parasites. I recently saw a patient who was very Blood Deficient and who went back to work without recover-ing properly from Malaria (see case study on page 122).

Dampness can also be a contributing factor to Blood Defi-ciency in the long term because it inhibits the digestive system and thus the body's ability to 'make' blood, so you should look at that entry as well (see page 116).

In my clinic, I see a lot of busy, high-achieving, over-worked, overstressed women who regularly push boundaries and very rarely rest. Unfortunately, that often means that they push their bodies beyond their limits and they can end up Blood Deficient. They may have a poor diet – not necessarily because of the quality of food they eat, but because they do not eat regularly and they don't eat enough. Factors that can contribute to becoming Blood Deficient include:

- regularly missing meals
- staying up late to work
- pushing yourself beyond your limits
- your body telling you to stop when your brain wants to go on

- suffering from an illness or nasty bug that's difficult to shift
- not resting properly after an illness
- a history of blood loss, including heavy periods.

Immediate steps to help deal with Blood Deficiency tendencies

First and foremost, I suggest you look at your eating patterns. I want you to eat regular meals in a relaxed environment – i.e. not on the run, in the car or out of a sandwich box on a train platform.

There is more information on good foods to nourish the blood in the section on diet (see page 167). A first-line treatment – as you probably already know from me – is chicken soup, but all soups are good. If you are a vegetarian, try the watercress and spinach soup on page 187. I also suggest leafy greens, or indeed any green vegetables, sprinkled with small black sesame seeds. Black or deep red foods are great – especially beans or berries. Seaweeds are also great for Blood Deficient types as well as anything high in protein.

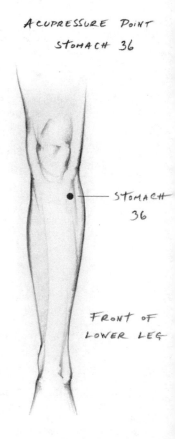

ACUPRESSURE POINT
STOMACH 36

STOMACH
36

FRONT OF
LOWER LEG

When someone is acutely Blood Deficient, I will also recommend that they see a Chinese herbalist. I also insist that a patient who is Blood Deficient should avoid alcohol at all costs. Alcohol creates Heat, which in turn consumes the Blood.

One other thing you could try yourself is applying moxibustion to acupressure point Stomach 36 (which is just under the knee – see diagram), because it helps assimilation, the digestion of food and therefore the manufacturing of Blood. (See page 82 for information on how to do this.)

Are you Heat?

I think that not only is the planet getting hotter, but so are those that inhabit it. And I don't mean that glibly. The traditional view of infertility in China was that it was all about Coldness, but this is not the experience of the modern-day practitioner. Today, I see far more people with Heat issues than Cold. This may be because of the highly polluted environment in which we live, which generates a lot of Heat. It may also be because of the way that we live. Alcohol, once again, is a contributing factor, as are stress and stimulants, such as coffee. Heat can also reflect unresolved emotional issues that have built up in the system. Common physical symptoms of Heat include:

- periods that come earlier than expected
- heavy periods
- bright red blood
- being prone to fevers – sometimes a fever with a period, fevers when you fall ill
- acne (which can also have a damp element, especially if the sores are weeping)
- lack of urine
- redness in the eyes
- inflammation in the body
- a strong thirst
- a red tongue
- rapid breathing
- dry stools.

Your type is most likely to be Heat if you agree with five to eight or more of the following statements:

- You like to have water by the side of the bed.
- You like to throw the covers off the bed.
- You often feel thirsty.

- You usually feel 'charged' and energetic.
- You have a hair-trigger temper.
- You react to things strongly.
- You often feel frustrated (this is also a strong indication of issues with the Liver, so refer to the section on Qi Stagnation, page 132).
- You find it difficult to relax.
- You are often agitated.
- You frequently get into spats with people around you.
- You binge (i.e. you do everything to the extreme – eat, drink, smoke, etc.).
- You often feel 'slighted' or 'burnt' by people.
- You lie awake at night churning over your difficulties.
- You wind yourself up into a state of rage.

NB: If you have low-grade symptoms of Heat, and suffer from night sweats, it is more likely that you are one of the advanced types that we call 'Yin Deficient.' For more information on this see page 129.

How does Heat affect your fertility?

According to Chinese medicine, too much Heat in the system can impact on the Blood. This combination is very significant in infertility patients and can cause implantation issues. Heat may create problems for the immune system, making it overactive and this may reject a developing embryo. The emotional agitation often caused by Heat may also hinder the process of implantation. It is important to keep calm. (See also Reckless Blood, page 138.)

COMBINATION TYPES

As I explained earlier, sometimes a patient can have symptoms of two types, which together produce a combined type. Actually, this is very common.

A good example is Damp/Heat. It is possible to reduce the amount of both dampening and heating foods by cutting out chocolate, alcohol, heavily spiced and fatty foods, such as curries, chickpeas and foods such as houmous. You can also introduce cooling and drying food such as bitter herbs and aduki beans, that drain dampness from the body.

What makes you Heat?

There are two main causes of Heat: one is a hot climate; the other is exposure to heat in the form of pollution and a 'heated-up' environment, so cities and areas of high industry. My patients tend to fall into the latter category. These are people who are always on the go, they never pay attention to their stress levels, they will shout whenever 'necessary'. They are the sharp-elbowed, pushy, 'get-out-of-my-way' types. At least twice a day, a Heat type will be at the centre of a frustrating altercation, usually involving voices being raised. Unresolved emotional issues are another cause of Heat.

That this high-octane way of communicating and living is on the increase is worrying. Those with intense Heat issues may find their rage harder to control, while the contributing factors continue to ratchet up their Heat levels.

In one of my dusty old Chinese teaching books there is a proverb. I paraphrase: 'When you think you are going to lose your temper, ask yourself: "What is more important, my anger or my health?"' The answer – for any of you who are wavering – is, of course, your health. So, please follow my recommendations.

CASE STUDY: HEAT

Becky came into my clinic, hot and flustered, and asked if she could open the window. She worked and played really hard and had a loud voice and a red face. Her skin was hot to touch.

We went through the consultation process, and as she was leaving, I said, 'You are a very, very good example of Heat – I'd hate, for example, to see you eat a lamb curry with a bottle of red wine followed by a coffee'. She looked amazed and said, 'That's exactly what I had for dinner last night!' Sometimes we are attracted to the things that do us harm.

Immediate steps to help deal with Heat tendencies

First and foremost, you should avoid:

- caffeine
- tobacco
- alcohol
- chocolate
- greasy foods
- sugar
- stimulants
- amphetamines or cocaine.

You have a responsibility both to yourself and to those around you. Heat can be a destructive condition for all concerned. If you think your issues with rage are getting out of control already, you need to seek professional help in addition to doing the cycles.

If your Heat is presenting as anger, you should also follow the instructions for (Liver) Qi Stagnation, as the two are often linked. If you feel it is impacting more on your digestion, you will need to pay attention to your diet.

In both cases, you need to learn how to manage stress, relax and harness your anger. You have to be able to calm down and break patterns of behaviour. Try meditation or yoga – they may be helpful.

Are you Stagnant?

The first point is that there are two types of Stagnation: Qi and Blood, and we'll look at each of these in turn.

Qi Stagnation

Qi Stagnation is shorthand for what is usually termed Liver Qi Stagnation. In Chinese medicine, the movement of Liver Qi – which, for the purposes of this book we will just call Qi – is essential for balanced emotions. Those who have deep-felt frustrations are often described as having Qi Stagnation.

Qi Stagnation is a real issue in fertility. As many as 70 per cent of the women who step into my clinic show signs of Qi Stagnation in the days before their menstrual bleed. The cases range from mild to severe.

The condition is usually caused by emotional frustration or a suppression of emotions, although the Pill and other medications can also contribute to it. You can see people with it all around you in everyday life: they are, for example, the drivers who get more than normally irritable when they are stuck in traffic, and who start shouting to release the frustration caused by the stuck Qi that has built up in their chests.

Qi plays an important role in the latter phase of the menstrual cycle, when the egg has not been fertilized and progesterone dips in order to trigger the uterus to shed the endometrial lining. At this point, Qi is responsible for helping the body adjust back to normal; so it's perhaps unsurprising that I see the condition in so many women who are anxious to conceive.

At some point in life, *everyone* suffers some symptoms of Qi Stagnation. Even that flickering irritation at being stuck in a traffic jam is a fleeting glimpse of Qi Stagnation.
Qi Stagnation can present as:
- gastritis, cholecystitis and Irritable Bowel Syndrome (IBS)
- PMS
- pelvic inflammatory disease (PID).

You may have issues with Qi Stagnation if you strongly agree with five to eight of the following statements:
- You sigh a lot.
- You feel irritable.
- You're prone to fluctuations in mood, from tearfulness to anger.
- You're indecisive.

- You feel frustrated.
- You frown a lot; you have a furrow between your brows.
- You can't finish projects.
- You can't move on.
- You feel uncomfortable in your own skin.
- You have random aches in your body.
- Your tongue has a mauve tinge.
- You feel uncomfortable after you eat.
- You bloat easily.
- Your breasts often feel swollen.
- Your periods are irregular.
- You have particular tenderness underneath your ribs.
- One bad thing happens after the other.
- You are out of control and can't get back on to an even keel.
- Your daily frustrations affect your sleep.
- You feel 'stuck in life', as if you're 'treading water' and not getting anywhere.

How does Qi Stagnation affect your fertility?
Stagnation is common in fertility because of the frustrations inherent in trying to get pregnant in the first place. And then of course, it can feed on itself. If the Qi is stagnant at the time of ovulation you may not successfully release an egg. Another potential problem is that the fertilized egg requires a free flow of Qi to enable it to travel down the Fallopian tube. If the Qi doesn't flow smoothly and there are contractions, the fertilized egg may arrive once the endometrium has already started to break down or at a stage that doesn't synchronize perfectly with implantation.

What makes you Qi Stagnated?
Unfortunately modern life itself is one of the biggest contributing factors in Stagnation. However, emotional issues or

baggage, current or from the past, can have an impact on your Qi and cause it to Stagnate.

Alcohol temporarily acts to move Qi Stagnation and acts as a cover for the existing emotional issue. The relief is short-lived, obviously, because alcohol cannot resolve the root of the problem and, ultimately, it ends up deepening it.

Qi Stagnation in its early stages isn't really a problem; it becomes one when the patient gets stuck in a rut and that then becomes their default setting for dealing with life in general.

Qi Stagnation that is left untreated often turns into Heat, which also plays havoc with the menstrual cycle. If you are concerned that you might be Stagnant with elements of Heat, try both diets and follow the exercise plans too (see pages 137 and 169).

Dealing with Qi Stagnation tendencies

There are two ways you can tackle Qi Stagnation: making yourself mentally more relaxed and changing your pace of life and the type of activities you participate in. Diet is also relevant.

Qi Stagnation responds very well to treatment. As it is very much an emotional blockage, rebalancing is largely on a psychological level; it's about outlook. So, it's not what happens to you, it's how you deal with it. This means repetitive therapy, meditation and a concerted effort to change patterns of behaviour. It involves being creative and changing the way you approach life in general. For patients with severe cases I recommend that they seek psychiatric help in addition to following my advice.

For immediate tips, see the list below. In the medium to long-term, it's a good idea to find activities where you feel you are positively releasing any pent-up frustration. A book club seems to be a popular option because it allows you to carve out time to read, but also to write up ideas and discuss them, which is good for the flow of Qi. Equally, going to a debate can help lift frustrations from your chest, but not if you have a tendency to get too het up.

Another thing that helps is organizing or sorting things out. This could be as simple as clearing out a messy kitchen drawer or colour-coding your knickers drawer, or more challenging – a full-on spring clean. The central point, however, is that it should feel enjoyable, not at all like a chore.

A Stagnated Qi also needs to get moving again, so in addition to the mental therapies, I recommend some exercise that gets you out and about and physically moving. I suggest a walk in the country, as this has the added benefit of being good time alone and helping you to work through ideas.

If you do these things regularly, throughout the month, it should lessen the impact on your premenstrual phase. The build-up won't be as bad and you won't have that need for a real outpouring any more. Here are some tips for emotional release:

- Be inventive with the way you choose to react to things (see the mental exercise below).
- Change the record – complaining keeps you in a rut.
- Lighten your load – an overambitious 'to-do' list can cause you to stall.
- Don't feel you have to 'challenge' everything.
- Use distraction – do something different, don't dwell. (This doesn't mean losing sight of your heart's desire; it's rearranging your mental outlook so that one issue doesn't cloud everything.)
- Don't put things off – the feeling of completing a project and moving on to something new is excellent for clearing Qi Stagnation.

Q&A

I am having difficulty working out my type as I have symptoms in all the categories.
This is common. Look for the main symptoms or the ones you have had more regularly and for longer. If you are unsure use the tongue to decide. It is a really good indicator and often reflects what you are needing at that moment. If it looks coated, follow Damp type, if red, follow Heat type etc.

- Use a different perspective. Take a step back or ask someone close to you to take a step back for you and give you an honest appraisal.
- Bounce ideas around with friends; freelancers are more prone to stuck Qi because they are not in an office or 'team' environment.
- Resolve emotionally difficult relationships.
- Shout: pretend you have a lost dog in the park and shout for him repetitively to release any stuck Qi in your chest.
- Sing, laugh and be a free spirit – don't take life so seriously.

For physical release try:
- going out for a brisk walk
- dancing
- swimming (but not during your period)
- playing sports – tennis, running, squash, etc.
- physically shaking off your problems (see box on page 136 and see qigong, pages 172–3).

And some dietary tips:
- Keep your liver clear – and by this I mean liver in the Western sense: cut out or at least cut right back on alcohol. Alcohol and Qi Stagnation is a lethal mix.
- On page 170, you will find recommendations for light, easily digestible foods, such as green and root vegetables, watercress, fennel and grains.)
- Add squash to my chicken soup recipe, along with coriander or dill.
- Fruit is good, but allow yourself time to digest your main meal before eating it. A grapefruit for breakfast, for example, would be excellent.
- Complex and over-rich meals should be avoided.
- Beware of 'comfort eating' – stay away from cakes, chocolate and ice creams. Avoid too much salt and sugar!

Blood Stagnation

This condition is linked to Qi Stagnation because it is the Qi's job to move the blood around the body, and there can be a knock-on effect on the blood if Qi stagnates. Blood Stagnation can have far more serious physical implications and some of the conditions associated with it may require surgery.

Blood Stagnation can present as:

- pain at the site of surgery
- broken veins and capillaries under the skin
- varicose veins
- fibroids
- endometriosis.

You may be Blood Stagnated if you agree with between five and eight of the following statements:

- You feel frustrated.
- You feel tired.
- You have a heavy, weighed-down, dragging feeling.
- You have stabbing pains in certain areas of your body.
- You bruise easily.
- You extremities – such as your feet – get cold.
- You get pins and needles.
- Your tongue is purple.
- There is a purple hue around your mouth.
- The veins underneath your tongue are swollen or distended.
- There are purple dots along your tongue.
- You have severe stabbing pain and blood clots when your period starts.

How does Blood Stagnation affect your fertility?

Blood Stagnation is a threat to fertility on a physical level be-cause if the blood isn't moving efficiently you can experience serious fertility problems such as endometriosis. Patients with this will often spot dark blood after their period. Another classic sign is when patients have had miscarriages or failed IVF cycles even though the embryos have been very good.

If the problem is deep-set, surgery is often needed. This is usually the case for the removal of fibroids, endometriosis and other conditions linked to Stagnant conditions.

What makes you Blood Stagnated?

Blood Stagnation develops from other conditions such as Cold and Damp, but localized Blood Stagnation can be a result of trauma and injury.

It is different from Qi Stagnation which, as we have seen, is usually triggered by an emotional issue. However, there is some overlap in the treatment, so do look at the advice above. As I have explained, Blood Stagnation is an advanced pathology and often requires a multi-disciplinary approach, some-

---

CHOOSE YOUR REACTION

Take what is widely acknowledged to be a frustrating situation, such as being in a traffic jam when you are late for an appointment, and think about how you would react. Remember – whatever you do, it's not going to change the situation. So, you may as well choose to practise remaining calm.

This is an easy – and quite fun – exercise that can help you learn how to take back control. Apply it whenever you feel that the rage is taking over and

that you are losing control.

Whenever you feel like immediately 'losing it', try a shrug-it-off gesture, by physically lifting and holding and then dropping and releasing your shoulders. Another physical letting-go gesture is to shake your hands as if drying them without a towel (see box on qigong and the shaking exercise, page 173).

The benefits of this are obvious whether you come from a Western or Eastern perspective.

times including surgery, and from a Chinese medicine point of view, herbal medicine too. Confusingly, Blood Stagnation can also be *caused* by surgery – a Caesarean section, for example; but in the case of a C-section straightforward acupuncture will improve pelvic blood flow.

Dealing with Blood Stagnation tendencies

I start treatment by trying to get the Qi moving, as Qi can move the Blood. Often, blood-clotting disorders in Western medicine fall into this category and are treated with blood thinners, such as aspirin or Heparin. Where surgery is involved, you will still need to address the underlying cause, so I'd strongly recommend that you follow the cycles to support the Western approach.

Although we see good results with the symptoms of Blood Stagnation through acupuncture, I also send my patients to see a herbalist and work closely with a gynaecologist. Two immediate recommendations are:

- abdominal massage.
- Daverick Leggett's[3] tea to help work on the movement of Qi. To prepare, simmer equal parts of cinnamon, ginger and tangerine peel in water until you have reduced the tea by a third, then drink.

Another food that is great for moving Blood is aubergine. However, aubergine should be avoided in the later half of the cycle if you are trying to conceive or in the very early stages of pregnancy because of its heavy moving effect on the blood in the uterus. In the Far East it is accepted that aubergine is avoided at this stage in the cycle and in the early weeks of pregnancy.

By now, you will be fully aware of your fertility type/s and ready to move on to the exciting bit – Part Two: The Menstrual Cycle. You can start it at any time, just find the chapter that is relevant to the stage you're at in your cycle: Chapter Four covers Days 1–5; Chapter Five, Days 6–13; Chapter Six, Day 14; Chapter Seven, Days 15–27.

Advanced conditions

Yin Deficiency

Yin Deficiency usually occurs in patients with severe Heat or in those who are seriously Blood Deficient. Yin is the cooling, moistening aspect of our bodies, the part that lubricates the 'engine' and stops us from seizing up.

An abundance of Yin will give rise to healthy, fertile secretions and a calm and grounded disposition. Like Blood Deficiency, the Yin Deficiency develops from overwork and/ or failure to recover properly from a prolonged illness, work-

RECKLESS BLOOD

When Heat is present over a period of time it begins to Heat the Blood – this results in what is called 'Reckless Blood' in Chinese medicine. The term amuses me: it suggests the Blood going out on a spending spree or driving really fast. What it actually refers to, however, is the Blood becoming Hot – we all know that feeling of something making our blood 'boil'.

In fertility, this feeling disrupts the menstrual cycle, causing irregular bleeding, and it can prevent the fertilized egg from implanting. I've seen this in women who spot bright red blood prior to the bleed, who have repeated miscarriages or IVF that fails at implantation. I've also seen it in women who appear to miscarry at the implantation stage. They may feel pregnant, but then their period will come – perhaps late – with bright red blood. I have seen some correlation with this condition and some Western medicine blood conditions, but this needs further research.

ing and playing hard and burning the candle at both ends – it is a real 'burnout' condition and I do, sadly, see it in clinic in some of the cases that are harder to treat.

Signs that Yin Deficiency has developed are what we call Five Palm Heat, which means the patient has heat or mild sweating in the palms of their hands, on the soles of their feet, and a feeling of heat in the centre of their chest. Symptoms include night sweats, feelings 'hot' in the afternoon and a tongue that is either without coating or has shiny patches without any coating. The skin is often dry and shows early signs of ageing and the patient is often highly strung and anxious.

The danger for a Yin Deficient woman who is receiving treatment for fertility is that they will produce little or no fertile cervical mucus. Their endometrium may fail to thicken and their follicles may not swell to reach maturity. In a man, Yin Deficiency manifests itself as scant and somewhat condensed sperm. This condition is harder to treat with lifestyle changes alone, although – obviously – heeding all the following will help:

- Absolutely don't drink coffee.
- Absolutely don't drink alcohol.
- Absolutely do not smoke.
- Take lots of rest – even time out from work if finances allow.
- Have early nights – no staying up late using the computer or watching TV.
- Eat lots of Yin-nourishing foods with every meal, such as apples, lemons, honey, eggs, tofu, seaweed, pork, pear, kidney beans, pineapple, and don't skip meals.

Note: Yin Deficient types also need to be careful on the fertility drug Clomid (see page 284).

IN A NUTSHELL: WHAT CAN YOU DO *NOW*?

- **Cold** Introduce some ginger to your diet; add it to food, try ginger tea.
- **Damp** Introduce aduki beans; try them in curries, soup or stews.
- **Blood Deficiency** Try seaweed or black sesame seeds; be adventurous.
- **Heat** Have a daily cup of fresh mint tea.

- **Yin Deficiency** Introduce more oily fish in your diet.
- **Qi Stagnation** Chop some coriander or dill into a soup or sprinkle on to a risotto.
- **Blood Stagnation** Try out some recipes that include aubergines.
- **Yang Deficiency** Avoid too much water.

Yin Deficiency and IVF

These types are often termed 'poor responders' in IVF, i.e. they don't produce many embryos. In this case, preparation is the key: do three to four months of IVF preparation, if your age allows.

I personally don't like to see women doing more that three IUI cycles with Clomid without a break of at least a month, because this drug dries the Yin fluids. Some of the consultants I work with will ask me if the patient is suitable for IUI based on my assessment of their energy and their Yin. Yin Deficient types find it hard to withstand the rigours of IVF, and the condition can actually often develop in women who have done lots of cycles (see Chapter Nine).

Immediate steps to help deal with Yin Deficiency tendencies

- Consult an acupuncturist.
- Consult a herbalist.
- Don't be in a hurry to rush from one thing to the next.
- Practise meditation and visualization (see pages 76

and 207). Your visualizations should include cooling, moistening imagery, such as water washing over the body, calming, soothing and repairing as it touches the skin.

Yang Deficiency

The primary function of Yang is to warm and transform – the opposite of Yin. The main symptoms of a Yang deficiency are those of a Cold type, but more extreme. A Yang Deficient patient may find their body is lacking in form – flabby – and it may feel cold and/or clammy to touch. Yang Deficient types may feel generally apathetic and sluggish with low energy.

In Chinese Medicine, these are all classic signs of infertility. If Cold presides for too long, it can damage the Yang of the body. Many activities damage the Yang – eating food straight from the fridge, drinking cold drinks with ice, swimming during the menstrual cycle and exposure to too much cold.

From a Western medical perspective, a Yang Deficient patient is sometimes found to be lacking in progesterone, which may lead to implantation failure in the 'follicular phase' – see page 218.

Sleep is vital here, so no matter what else you do, make sure you rest. Other key factors are diet, Moxibustion, herbal medicine (or progesterone).

Infertility patients who are Kidney Yang Deficient do quite well on Clomid since the warming effect of this drug improves their luteal phase – for more on this, see Chapter Eight.

Q&A
Which of the types has the biggest effect on fertility?
It is more a case of how deeply set the problem is. So someone may have relatively mild Blood Deficient symptoms which improve quickly, or they can have severe symptoms which will take much longer. Generally Qi stagnation is easier to treat, if the patient really takes on board the mind's involvement. Yin Deficiency (Chapter Three) is generally considered a more advance condition and therefore harder to treat.

Part II
THE BABY-
MAKING PLAN

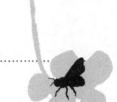

Chapter Four

Days 1–5: Menstruation

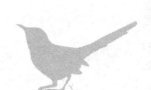

Your menstrual cycle can affect your mood, voice, behaviour, outlook on life and even whether men see you as attractive or not. Equally, it is affected by your mood, grief, ill health, bad diet, frequent travel and changes in time zone.

This and the following three chapters deal exclusively with your cycle – in my baby-making plan you'll find recommendations for diet and exercise, tips for building mental strength and descriptions of what is going on from both the Western and Chinese medicine points of view.

My aim is to put you back in touch with your natural cycle and the phases within it, making you feel healthy and more in control and showing you that you do have choices when it comes to trying to conceive a healthy baby. If I can help you balance your body and mind throughout your menstrual cycle, you have a good chance of getting healthy and getting pregnant. I call it 'fine-tuning the engine'. In Chapter Three, you will have established which type/s you are according to Chinese medicine, and now I want you to follow the advice for that type throughout your menstrual cycle.

You'll find a description of exactly what is going on in your body at each stage. I urge you to try to visualize each stage as it happens – your healthy eggs ripening, your endometrium (womb lining) building up, the egg releasing from the follicle and then implanting. As you read the descriptions, imagine your body effortlessly and beautifully completing each phase.

How to use the twenty-eight-day plan

The word menstrual comes from the Latin menses, which comes from the Greek word for moon, mene. The average menstrual cycle is around twenty-eight days long (although anything from twenty-seven to thirty-two days is generally considered acceptable), with ovulation occurring on Day 14. There are three distinct phases: the infertile period of menstruation, then the fertile period, during which we ovulate, followed by another infertile period of two weeks, during which a fertilized egg will embed in the uterus.

Your 'period' will occur fourteen days after ovulation, which happens to be in the middle if your cycle is twenty-eight days long. If your cycle is, say, thirty-two days long, calculate your fertile time by counting backwards from the first day of your period (you will ovulate on Day 18, so your fertile time is between Days 14 and 18).

My plan is set to a twenty-eight-day cycle, but it is perfectly adaptable to a cycle of any length. This chapter and Chapter Five deal with your period and the week before ovulation. If your cycle is longer than twenty-eight days, you'll need to spend more time following the advice either on the period (if your period is longer than five days) or the phase after your period (if this is where you are accumulating days in your cycle).

Those of you who have a shorter cycle may have to skip a few days. So, if your period is shorter than five days, drop a few days in this chapter; if your period is five days, but you ovulate on Day 8, cut some days from Chapter Five.

Everyone should follow Chapter Six, which deals with ovulation and Chapter Seven, which covers the two weeks after that. Most women menstruate two weeks after ovulation.

Embracing your period

First, I am going to urge you to shake off any prejudices you have about your period. Women often arrive at my clinic for the first time referring to their period as 'the curse' (an allusion to the curse of Eve). It seems we have had it drilled into us from an early age that this is one of many burdens we women bear, and that a bad, painful period is some sort of punishment.

In some religions, women were and are considered 'impure' or 'unclean' during menstruation and, historically, were separated from the rest of the group. There are examples where menstruating women were forbidden to touch, among other things, food, wildlife and men. Perhaps, unsurprisingly, this idea of a 'curse' has been passed down through the generations as a thing of shame.[2]

For modern women, the arrival of their period is popularly associated with all things unattractive: a spotty complexion, bloated abdomen, sore breasts, a tendency to cry, as well as cravings for unhealthy sugar-laden foods such as cakes and chocolate. Our periods are, throughout our lives, supposed to be accompanied by

> **Q&A**
> *I have bad period pains which are soothed by a hot-water bottle, and there are lots of clots, what is your advice?* This sounds like a combined pattern. You have an element of Cold (because you feel better with warmth) which has probably existed for sometime and has caused the Blood to stagnate. You need to follow the advice for Cold types and include some mild exercise during your period to help move the Blood. Do not get cold or go swimming as this will make the problem worse. Eat aubergines and cooked foods while you have your period.

aches, pains, regular doses of strong painkillers and a fair amount of complaining. Periods are, unfortunately, political. (But then so is just about everything else to do with fertility, pregnancy, childbirth, breastfeeding and child-rearing!)

So, I want you to take a deep breath now, and completely revolutionize the way in which you view your period. This may take real effort, but for conception, you need to try. I want you to feel in tune with your cycle; and that includes menstruation. I'm not suggesting that you go outside and wave your sanitary towels in the street, but I do want you to reclaim your period mentally.

Your period is your inner guide. It gives you a chance to enhance your awareness and learn more about your health and fertility. It is the symbol of a new beginning; trying to cut it out is rather like trying to get rid of Monday. So, Day One heralds the beginning of the next cycle. Hormones are released in the pituitary gland in the brain that stimulate the ten to fifty maturing eggs, one of which will be released during ovulation around fourteen days later. Think of it as a fresh start: another month in which to get healthy. In clinic, we view this as the optimum time to treat certain conditions, especially those that benefit from the movement of Blood. For some women, it can be an emotionally difficult time, but most are prepared to turn it into one of opportunity.

Often, the same women who initially viewed their period as the curse, ultimately embrace it as a time that has equal importance to ovulation. 'Curse or cure?' a patient recently asked me, after successfully balancing her cycle. She answered: 'I think the latter.'

Q&A

I find my mood is very low on the day my period arrives and I feel very tearful and emotional. What can I do?

Follow the advice for Qi Stagnant types and address your emotional needs throughout the months. Stress relief and meditation are very important to help you to feel in control of your mood. I do think that issues that arise with the period are areas we need to address in our lives so it is important not to ignore them. Make sure you put time aside for yourself.

Understanding your cycle

Fertility 'issues' can be relatively simple. One third of the couples I see discover in our chats that they are not having enough sex, or that they are not having enough sex at the right time. (See page 182 for more on the right kind of sex at the right time.) On the whole, I am not surprised: we tend to spend the first part of our lives trying to avoid pregnancy at all costs (ironically, probably at the time in our life when we are having the most sex); then we spend the next part trying to have enough sex, but failing to fit it around busy lives and sometimes missing the most fertile times.

Understanding the precise mechanisms of your cycle can help you visualize how your hormones, your body and your reproductive system work – especially if you go on to have issues conceiving. So I am going to tell you all about the reproductive system. Even if you think you know it all already, bear with me. We are going to start with the basics.

The female reproductive system
Ovaries
Most women have two functioning ovaries, one on the left and one on the right of their uterus. Each ovary is the size of a walnut, and this is where eggs are produced, stored (in frond-like follicles in the ovarian wall) and released once every cycle at the time we call ovulation (we deal with this in Chapter Six).

The egg (ovum)
A baby girl is born with between 1 and 2 million potential eggs (also called oocytes). These are found in fluid cavities called follicles on the ovarian wall. Over the years of a female's life – from birth until the menopause – these egg cells are gradually depleted, so that by puberty, the number has

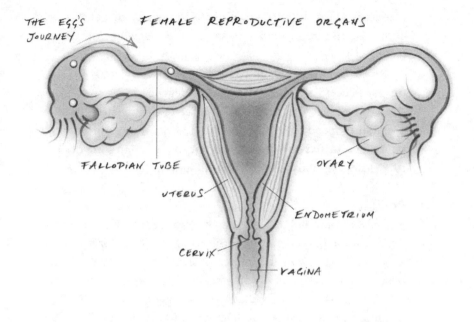

THE EGG'S JOURNEY — FEMALE REPRODUCTIVE ORGANS

FALLOPIAN TUBE

UTERUS

CERVIX

OVARY

ENDOMETRIUM

VAGINA

dipped to around 300,000. A fraction of those – around four to five hundred – will mature into eggs, one by one, and be released in the menstrual cycles that occur from puberty until the menopause.

As your menstrual cycle moves towards the fertile period, between ten and fifty oocytes begin to mature and usually one (occasionally more) will rise to the top of the follicle and be released into the Fallopian tube. This matured egg is the size of a pinhead.

The egg moves into the Fallopian tube where, if it meets a sperm, it may be fertilized. If a sperm penetrates the surface of the egg, the egg will immediately form an extra membrane to prevent other sperm from penetrating.

As the oocytes are not subject to any of the cellular repair processes that can occur with other cells in our bodies, as a woman gets older, the likelihood of damage to these egg cells increases. (This, in turn, increases the chance of genetic or chromosomal abnormality if any of these eggs go on to be fertilized.)

As a woman gets closer to the menopause, the body speeds up the process by which these eggs degenerate. It may also start releasing more than one egg per cycle. Eventually, the body stops producing mature, viable eggs. Once the menopause has started and the fertile stage of a woman's life draws to a close, the body ceases egg production.

Follicles

The release of follicle-stimulating hormone (FSH) and luteinizing hormone (LH) from the pituitary gland in the brain, triggers the maturity of a number of eggs in the ovaries. The protective follicles then produce an increasing amount of the hormone oestrogen, which, in turn, triggers the production of mucus in the cervix (see Chapter Five). This mucus is designed to help sperm swim towards – and eventually reach – the released egg. As the mid-cycle approaches (see Chapters Five and Six), the follicle ruptures allowing the egg to be released into the Fallopian tube.

Fallopian tubes

The Fallopian tubes link the ovaries to the uterus and are covered by tiny hairs that help move the egg down to meet the strong-swimming sperm. The sperm penetrates the egg, and once it reaches its nucleus, the two fuse to form one single cell – the first cell of new life, called the zygote (see Chapter Seven).

The single cell divides and these cells continue to divide as the mass (or 'morula') travels towards the uterus. It takes a further four days to arrive, becoming, as it does so, a 'blastocyst'.

The uterus

The uterus is the womb – your egg's destination following its release from the follicle and journey down the Fallopian tube. Before conception, your uterus is the size of a plum, or your fist. If you conceive, it will rapidly expand with the baby and will have doubled in size by seven weeks.

In ideal conditions, the endometrium (uterine wall) will be 9mm thick and soft and ready for the blastocyst's arrival and implantation at around nine days after fertilization. As you will learn in my plan, there is a lot you can do to help build up a thick, receptive endometrium ripe for implantation.

Once it is embedded, the blastocycst connects with your bloodstream through hair-like cells on its surface and absorbs the nutrients in your system. This blastocyst becomes the embryo, evolving at three months into a foetus.

If the egg is not fertilized, the endometrial lining is shed and you experience this as the blood during menstruation. If the egg is fertilized, but does not properly embed, it is classed as a very early miscarriage. In most cases, you will not even be aware that conception has occurred.

Hormones

The hormones produced during each stage of your menstrual cycle allow your body to go through the magical processes that put each cog in motion and make you ripe for conception and will ultimately enable you to conceive.

These hormones are extremely important and can be disturbed and upset by physical and emotional imbalance. This can not only affect your cycle, but also conception. Balanced hormones are vital for good fertility.

Male reproductive system
Sperm
Unlike the egg's cells, sperm – or spermatozoa – are continuously

produced in an almost daily process of renewal throughout a
man's life. In any one ejaculation, between 1 and 400 million
sperm are released.

Sperm are often compared to tadpoles in shape, but they
are tiny (just 0.05mm long) and a single sperm cell is the
smallest cell in the human body; their tails are hundreds of
times thinner than a human hair.

There are 'male' (Y) and 'female' (X) sperm cells – the egg
is always an X chromosome – and they carry twenty-three of
the chromosomes that, combined with the twenty-three chromosomes of the egg, will create the genetic blueprint of the
next generation.

Received wisdom tells that male sperm swim faster, but

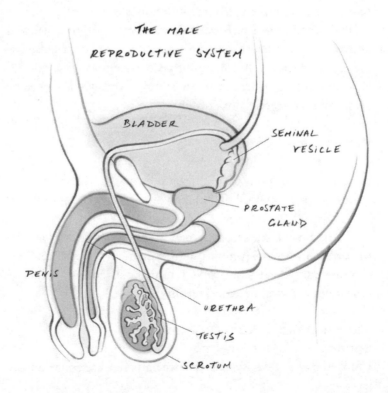

don't live as long as female sperm – hence the idea that if you have sex closer to ovulation you are more likely to conceive a boy, but if you have sex a couple of days before ovulation, you are more likely to conceive a girl. (This is by no means an exact science.)

Sperm are manufactured in the testicles, then they move to the back of the testes where they mature over a few days. As sperm turn over frequently, regular ejaculation can have a direct effect on keeping them healthy. General health, therefore, can impact on the sperm. For more on sperm, see Chapter One (page 46) and the Male Cycle (page 196).

The body naturally regulates the temperature at which sperm is kept. The optimum temperature is several degrees lower than body temperature. Sperm can be damaged if the scrotum gets too cold – hence the body pulls the testicles towards the heat of the body. Equally, sperm can be damaged by too much heat: chefs are said to have an increased chance of damage to their sperm because they work in an environment where intense heat is directed below waist height.

Other causes of too much heat could be tight clothing, laptops that are used – as their name suggests – on the lap and even mobile phones that are kept in trouser pockets.

Is the engine working?

As levels of oestrogen and progesterone drop, the endometrial lining in the uterus begins to fall away, signaling the start of your period. At the same time, a number of eggs ripen in the ovary, ready for one to be released later in the cycle. In Chinese medicine this is the follicular or 'Yin phase'.

Observing the blood flow during your period
Mark in your diary Day One. If you start in the late afternoon

or evening, the following day is considered Day One.

Ideally, menstruation begins with a light flow of red blood, followed by the main flow, which is a little heavier, within twenty-four hours. Your period should be without clots, without pain and it should last an average of four to five days.

WHY I BELIEVE IN A FOUR-MONTH PRE-CONCEPTION BABY-MAKING PLAN

For a long time, I worked with a three-month pre-conception preparation cycle which was very successful. Part of the thinking behind it was that sperm take seventy-two to eighty-six days to develop in a process called spermatogenesis, and I still advocate a three-month plan for men. After consulting with both patients and colleagues, however, I decided that four months was a better preparation period for women, time and age allowing. This was for two reasons.

First of all, four months (or 120 days) is the time it takes for the eggs to become mature in the ovaries. This process is called folliculogenesis. I decided that working with the body's natural cycle would be a better way of achieving optimum fertility health.

This was backed up by anecdotal evidence from patients who chose to work with a four-month cycle. They had a much higher rate of positive outcomes and reported feeling even better in their 'overall wellbeing'.

Second, I have always believed that most fertility journeys are very linear. Often women have no cohesive plan and when things don't happen as they expect, they feel out of control. This is why a plan of action is good: it really helps to manage the stress and makes the process feel more fun and enjoyable.

In my practice, I put my patients into a cycle of treatment that has a beginning, a middle and an end: this lasts four months. It is far more reassuring than the stop-start lurching-from-period-to-ovulation approach that distresses so many women who are trying to conceive. During this preparation time they are not actively trying to conceive, but are thinking about 'fertility'. I want them to get away from the idea that with every passing month they are moving further from their dream of having a baby, and, by spending time concentrating on 'fertility', getting healthy and dealing with minor or major obstacles, they are gently moving towards their goal of a healthy conception.

There should be no spotting after your period has finished. If, however, it doesn't fit this description, don't worry; follow the advice below and you should find that your cycle starts to match the 'ideal' within a couple of months.

If this is your first cycle, it is particularly vital to make a note of what is happening in your diary, when things occur and how you feel, so that you can chart the changes in subsequent cycles. This is a really important time because this is when you are going to see the changes manifest and, often, the menstrual cycle is where this happens first.

If this is your second cycle, you may already be experiencing some changes. The flow may have improved and become closer to the ideal, the pain might have eased or your mood may have improved. You are doing really well. Keep going! (Patients who suffered from PMT and have followed this plan say that after a couple of efforts their period just arrived, with no symptoms at all.)

If this is your third or fourth cycle, you may have noticed a real change in your symptoms by now. The vast majority of my patients have an enormous sense of achievement at this stage. They have actually made a difference to the way they look and feel (it's very empowering!) and they really start to understand the power of Chinese medicine – it wins even the most hardened sceptics around.

Menstrual problems

- **Amenorrhoea** (no periods) This can be caused by Blood Deficiency, Blood Stagnation or Damp.
- **Metrorrhagia** (heavy or prolonged periods) This can be caused by Heat or Blood Stagnation (and Qi Deficiency).
- **Dysmenorrhoea** (painful periods) This can be caused by any of the conditions: Cold, Damp/Heat, Blood Deficiency or Qi and Blood Stagnation.

155

YOUR MENSTRUAL CYCLE

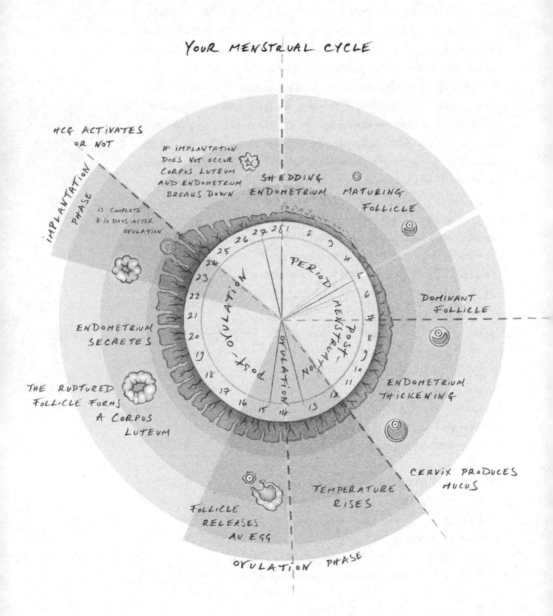

HCG ACTIVATES OR NOT

IF IMPLANTATION DOES NOT OCCUR CORPUS LUTEUM AND ENDOMETRIUM BREAKS DOWN

SHEDDING ENDOMETRIUM

MATURING FOLLICLE

IMPLANTATION PHASE

IS COMPLETE 8-10 DAYS AFTER OVULATION

PERIOD

POST-OVULATION

DOMINANT FOLLICLE

ENDOMETRIUM SECRETES

OVULATION

MENSTRUATION

POST-MENSTRUATION

ENDOMETRIUM THICKENING

THE RUPTURED FOLLICLE FORMS A CORPUS LUTEUM

CERVIX PRODUCES MUCUS

FOLLICLE RELEASES AN EGG

TEMPERATURE RISES

OVULATION PHASE

Most women have an inkling when something is not quite right. How they respond to that, however, is crucial. Patients will sometimes tell me: 'I went travelling for a year and didn't have any periods all that time; it was great!' Yet periods are central to the reproductive process, and mentally suppressing them at times when they would be inconvenient can have a knock-on negative impact when it comes to wanting to conceive.

This is why I urge you to embrace the *entire* menstrual cycle. Your mind can have a phenomenal effect on your body: don't send mixed messages to your uterus!

Is the fuel good?

For everyone for Days 1–5

- Ideally you shouldn't use tampons, but I realize this can be difficult, so try to limit your use and don't use them at night.
- Refrain from sex during your period (especially if you are Blood Stagnant).
- Don't swim during your period.
- Use acupressure – the recommended points are listed below under type.
- I advocate rest: go to bed early as often as possible for these five days.
- Bergamot, chamomile and cypress oils are great for menstrual pain. Use them neat in the bath or dilute in a carrier oil for massage – almond oil is good.
- This is a time of emotional quiet – don't get embroiled in rows or upheaval.
- This is also a time of renewal and clarity of vision – invest time in ideas, plans and being creative.

Diet

Let me start by saying that we're not talking here about *diet* in the calorie-counting, restrictive-eating sense. It is as much about *introducing* the foods to help your type as it is about eliminating those that are contributing positively to your condition. I need you to look after and to nourish yourself, not starve. The advice and lists below are a means of offering you foods that will help your type. However, I want to reduce the stresses in your life, and these lists should not in any way bring you more stress, so just do what you can and enjoy the process – this is not a punishment!

If you find yourself in a situation where you are faced with foods on your 'avoid' list, allow yourself to enjoy something 'naughty', then counter it with something on your recommended list. Remember, Chinese medicine is all about balance. As you get healthier and happier, so your body will work better.

The lists for your store cupboard (below) are designed to empower you. Food in Chinese medicine is essential, pleasurable and medicinal, so your kitchen will play a large part in the plan to build up your health. Heart and hearth co-exist: by eating well you will nourish your Heart, which will in turn help to create the environment of vitality that you need for a healthy conception. In Chinese medicine there is a powerful saying: 'The Heart opens the Womb'.

Diet is also a great way to shift the emphasis placed on conception back on to the general idea of fertility: you are looking after yourself in order to improve your overall fertility.

Exercise

Many of you will have an existing exercise routine and you may well want to stick to that. May I suggest, however, that you also try both the qigong and the yoga sequences at the end of this chapter. These have been designed with this phase of the menstrual cycle in mind, and I want to encourage you to get into the zone on every level. However, they are also enjoyable – about relaxation and gentle stretches, not strenuous and exhausting working out. Again, it's all in the plan to make you feel good about yourself, which is very much part of the preparation for conception.

Advice for Cold types

My patients who have a tendency towards Cold often experience quite severe aches and pains around the time of their period and need warmth to relieve these. This warmth can come from several sources, including:

- a warm bath with essential oils such as bergamot and jasmine
- yoga, Pilates and exercises that involve stretching
- moxibustion (wave the smouldering moxa stick over your lower abdomen)
- yoga (see below for poses that help pain)
- a hot-water bottle
- the Womb Warmer (see page 81).

Diet

To help with a Cold condition try:

- ginger tea, cinnamon tea, thyme tea (see below)
- ginger and garlic added to the chicken soup recipe.

In addition, avoid:

- eating food straight from the fridge; let it warm to room temperature first
- eating raw foods, as far as possible
- drinking cold water, as it is harder to absorb; drink it at room temperature.

RECIPES FOR THOSE WITH COLD CONDITIONS

Quinoa and Thyme Salad
(Summer)

To make the quinoa, simply take 3 parts water to 1 part grain. Put the quinoa in a saucepan, add sprigs of fresh thyme, cover with the water, perhaps add a dash of marigold stock powder or Maldon salt, then bring to the boil, reduce to a simmer and cover. Simmer until all the water has been absorbed. When cooked and cooled, gently strip the softened thyme leaves and remove their stems. Toss the quinoa with toasted walnuts and fresh torn basil leaves, add cherry tomatoes, celery, spring onion and any vegetables of your choice, then drizzle with a vinaigrette made with crushed garlic and lemon juice.

Jani's Lamb Shank Stew with Rosemary *(Winter)*

Serves 2
2–3 lamb shanks
1 clove garlic, crushed
dash of olive oil
240ml stock
1 tsp Dijon mustard
a couple of glugs of red wine
carrot
4 large sprigs rosemary
sweet potatoes
2 bay leaves
celery
salt and pepper
leeks
fresh chopped parsley
onions
steamed green beans and
1 large tin chopped tomatoes
mashed potatoes, to serve

1. Rub the shanks (preferably from the butcher) with the olive oil and Dijon mustard and place in a roasting pan. Cook uncovered in a hot oven (200°C/400°F/gas mark 6) and brown for 10 minutes. This will help to sear the juices into the meat.

2. Meanwhile cut the vegetables into large chunks. Remove the pan from the oven and fill with the vegetables. In a separate bowl, mix the chopped tomatoes, garlic, stock and red wine. Pour this over the lamb and vegetables, then stuff the sprigs of fresh rosemary into the juices around the lamb. Add bay leaves and salt and pepper to taste.

3. Lower the oven to 140°C/275°F/gas mark 1 and slow cook the lamb for up to 4 hours. When you are just about ready to serve, steam some green beans. Then remove the lamb shanks from the oven. Take the shanks out of the stew, peel the meat off the bones and place the tender meat back into the stew. Add the steamed beans and some chopped parsley and serve with mashed potatoes. Cooking meat on the bone will nourish the broth with the marrow from the bones. This is very beneficial to the blood and to the Qi too.

Cold store cupboard

I think it's a good idea to stock your cupboard with the types of food that you will be eating over the next few cycles. These will be warming and stimulating foods and should increase your metabolism as well as your libido:

- Cinnamon, thyme, fenugreek
- Fennel (good for period pain and also to help regulate the menstrual cycle)
- Fennel seeds
- Quinoa (recommended for any woman trying to conceive)
- Sprouting fenugreek seeds – you can add these to sandwiches
- Black pepper
- Root vegetables, such as pumpkin, squash, turnip, sweet potato

Thyme tea

Thyme has a host of properties that are good for the female reproductive system, specifically relieving period pain and treating infections (including thrush). Take a handful of fresh thyme, stuff it into the teapot, steep for 5–7 minutes, then drink hot or cold. This is an excellent immune system builder and should be taken in large doses at the first sign of a cold or chesty infection. Good for coughs.

Coriander tea

Coriander drinks were made at weddings in the Middle Ages as an aphrodisiac and drunk in the *Arabian Nights* as a cure for impotence. It is good for low libido and can also be used to relieve period pain in all but Heat types. Dry-pan roast the coriander seeds over a low to medium heat. Leave them to cool and then steep in water. Drain for tea.

Advice for Damp types

Many people in the UK have a tendency to Damp, due to the predominantly damp climate, and this predisposition is exacerbated by modern life: we spend a lot of time sitting (at desks, in cars, on the sofa) and many of us get to the end of the day without enough stretching movement or vigorous exercise. Our food is highly processed, high in sugar, fat and preserving agents. We eat less seasonal food and less fresh wholefoods. Wheat and dairy are two of the biggest villains when it comes to causing Damp. And medicines such as antibiotics, steroids and the birth-control pill don't help.

Damp is often found in combination with either Cold or Heat, so check these conditions too. During Days 1–5 of your menstrual cycle, certain conditions related to Damp/Heat may flare up. These include: acne, bacterial infection, irritable bowel syndrome (IBS), hives and herpes.

Exercise

Exercise is essential for a Damp condition to oxygenate the body. Yoga and Pilates are excellent for this because they stretch the muscles both lengthways and across their fibres, which helps to eliminate Dampness from the muscles. All forms of movement are beneficial. Aim to incorporate a small amount of exercise into each day – the aim is to keep things moving.

Diet

Dampening food is everywhere, so you may have to work a little harder than, say, someone with just a Heat condition, when choosing your food. The good news is that you will feel so much better once you start to eliminate Dampening foods from your diet and will significantly improve your chances of conceiving.

Avoid:
- raw foods – according to climate and season; so, don't eat salads in winter
- cold foods – room temperature or warmer is best
- refined foods
- highly processed foods
- saturated fats
- hydrogenated oils
- pork and rich meats (any meat with a high fat content)
- chemically treated foods
- glutinous foods
- too much soya
- non-organic meats
- non-organic eggs
- farmed fish
- excess salt
- sugars and sweeteners
- wheat
- yeasts/anything fermented (wine and beer)
- any juice from concentrate, especially tomato and orange
- tomato concentrate (purée)
- bananas
- peanuts
- oily nuts and seeds (except pumpkin, sunflower, walnut and almonds which are less congesting)
- ice cream
- cow's milk.

In addition, don't:
- reheat food more than once
- eat too many ingredients in one meal
- eat late in the evening
- overeat
- eat too fast

- eat while working or watching TV
- swallow without properly chewing
- drink too much water with your food – and sip, don't gulp.

When it comes to eating out, whether at restaurants – which do tend to have Damp-forming menus, unfortunately – or at someone's house, try not to be too precious. There is a lot of good in being fed by someone else and in not having to wash up afterwards. So enjoy the food and draw benefit from the situation. Once back in your own kitchen, however, seek to balance things out and be doubly conscious of avoiding Dampening foods.

Damp and dairy

'Cow's milk for butter, sheep's milk for cheese, goat's milk for drinking' – this is the advice of many a nutritionist, stretching back centuries. Cow's milk is particularly Dampening but naturally soured products such as yoghurt, crème fraîche, kefir (a fermented milk drink) and buttermilk are more easily digested than other forms of cow's dairy. Ice cream is not only Damp forming because of the cow's milk, but also due to the very high levels of sugar and, to top it all off, the very cold nature of this food renders it doubly difficult to digest. Steer well clear.

Try the following dairy substitutes:

- Almond milk (relieves tension and spasm and is good for period pain)
- Rice milk – such as Rice Dream
- Oat milk
- Soya – I don't recommend soya milk, but fermented soya products – such as tofu, tempeh, miso and soy sauce – are good, as they are much easier to digest.

Damp and wheat

Wheat can cause bloating, gas, stomach pain, indigestion and excessive mucus in a Damp condition, so it is best avoided. Many people who cannot tolerate processed-flour products do well with bulgur wheat, sprouted wheat and wheatgerm. These are wholegrain wheat products that deliver the full nourishment of wheat, often without the difficulties that processed wheat can present for a Damp condition.

Damp store cupboard

The following foods resolve Damp and are great to keep in your store cupboard:

- Aduki beans
- Alfalfa
- Anchovy
- Barley
- Button mushrooms
- Celery
- Corn
- Garlic
- Green tea
- Horseradish
- Jasmine tea
- Kidney beans
- Kohlrabi
- Lemon
- Mackerel
- Marjoram
- Mustard leaf
- Onion
- Parsley
- Pumpkin
- Radish
- Rye
- Spring onion
- Turnip

Advice for Blood Deficient types

There is one word to describe what Blood Deficient types should be doing on Days 1–5 of their cycle: resting. You need to rest, both mentally and physically. As corny as it sounds, you need some 'you' time. This is the week to crack open a new DVD box set, start a new novel or catch up on some movies.

I would prefer that you did no exercise; but if you must, try some breathing exercises and light yoga stretches.

Nettle Soup

Pick your own fresh nettles: find a place away from traffic fumes and where dogs will not have taken a pee! Wear rubber gloves, and using a carrier bag, only pick the tender nettle tops (the top six to eight leaves of fresh, new plants, about 30–45cm high; if they are in flower, they are too old). When you cook or steep the nettles the stingers will droop and no longer sting. They are too fine to sting through rubber gloves.

Serves 2
A knob of butter
1 large onion, chopped
2 cloves garlic, chopped
2 large potatoes, finely chopped
1.2 litres fresh young nettle tops (gently pack them into a measuring jug)
1.2–1.8 litres chicken or vegetable stock
fresh chopped parsley
dash of lemon juice
nutmeg
black pepper

1. Sauté the garlic and onion in butter, then add the chopped potato. Toss until the potatoes are well coated. Add the young nettle tops and add the chicken or vegetable stock. Bring it all to the boil and then gently simmer for 20 minutes.

2. Season with fresh chopped parsley and add the lemon juice and a grating of nutmeg, as well as plenty of freshly ground black pepper.

Orange and Prune Blood Builder

This is great for building the blood, and for relieving constipation. The vitamin C in the oranges encourages the absorption of iron from the prunes.

6 stoned prunes (tinned are best; avoid anything with added sugar)
2 large oranges (enough to make 80–120ml juice)
1 heaped spoonful live yoghurt (sheep and goat's yoghurt is more digestible than cow's)
ground cinnamon, to taste

1. Blend all the ingredients together as a smoothie.

Blood Deficient types should try:
- Spring onion essential oils in the bath, especially cardamom
- acupressure on Stomach 36 (see page 125) will help build Blood
- moxibustion on Stomach 36
- keeping things simple
- being sure to nourish, nourish, nourish
- chicken soup
- dandelion tea and nettle tea
- wheatgrass shots
- floradix – iron and vitamin liquid formula, available at health food shops.

Remember also that your memory is not great, so watch you don't leave the keys in the front door and jot down anything that is important on a list!

Diet

A lot of foods are good for nourishing the Blood, so you have a more interesting cycle ahead of you than those with a Damp condition, for example. Nonetheless there are a couple of things to watch. Avoid:
- sugar
- alcohol
- stimulants, such as coffee.

Blood Deficient store cupboard

Keep the following in your store cupboard:
- Black beans
- Black sesame seeds
- Blackcurrants
- Beetroot
- Carrots
- Cherries
- Dates
- Eggs
- Figs
- Grains
- Greens – especially dark, leafy ones
- Meat
- Seaweed

Also:
- Dandelion leaves and beetroot leaves: both are lovely in summer salads, especially when they are picked young.
- Wheatgerm, oat, bran and molasses: used in a muffin recipe, these make a nourishing blood-building snack to have at work or as part of a good breakfast.

Advice for Heat types

Heat types will often experience heavy menstrual bleeding. The actual act of menstruation itself drains the body of some Heat and helps relieve symptoms somewhat.

BONES

The Chinese believe in the power of 'like feeding like'. They believe that one of the best ways to nourish Blood and Qi Deficiency is with foods made with bone marrow. This will help your body to build its own reservoirs to power your physiology. In China, stock from marrow is said to 'promote growth and development' as it is full of omega 3s.

If you are cooking soups, stews or casseroles use meat on the bone, and to get the best value from the marrow, cook from raw. When roasting be sure to utilize the precious juices from the meat; these are the most beneficial part of the roast, as the juice is imbibed with the marrow. When cooking meat in a sauce the same applies; it is not the flesh that will give you the most strength but the juices.

There is a recipe for chicken stock on page 50. This forms the base for chicken – or any other – soup, and can also be used in stews and casseroles and to cook grains (such as rice, couscous, bulgur wheat, quinoa or millet); it will give you the benefits of added flavour, as well boosting the nutritional value of the grains.

A beef casserole made with root vegetables and seasoned with garlic and marjoram will strengthen both the Qi and the Blood. Slow cooking increases digestibility.

To alleviate problems associated with Heat try:
- baths with essential oils – chamomile, cypress, geranium and Rose are my favourites.
- peppermint tea or cool water with lemon and honey.
- ten minutes of acupressure on Spleen 10 page 225.
- no exercise on Days 1–5 (unless you are very used to it)
- keeping a cool pad in the fridge in case of migraines
- meditation (see page 76).

In addition, you should avoid:
- caffeine
- alcohol.

Diet

Raw foods are good for patients with a lot of Heat, such as salads in summer. Leafy greens, beans and pulses, whole grains, dried fruits, seeds and nuts, seaweeds and fresh fish are also great.

Miso soup is a staple in Japanese diets and it's great for Heat types; the ingredients are now readily available in most supermarkets and all good health-food shops.

Make fruit salads using fruits on the list below to cool down your system. I always advise patients to eat fruit on its own and at least 20 minutes before or after anything else.

Heating foods, such as curries and greasy foods should be avoided.

Heat store cupboard

Keep the following in your store cupboard:
- Apples
- Asparagus
- Cheese
- Duck
- Eggs
- Peas
- Pineapple
- Pomegranate
- Pork
- Seaweed

- Honey
- Kidney beans
- Lemons
- Malt
- Mangoes
- Milk
- Parsley
- Pears

- Sesame seeds
- Shellfish
- Spelt
- String beans
- Tomatoes
- Tofu
- Watermelon
- Yam

Note: while wheat is bad for those with a Damp condition, it is cooling in nature and is therefore beneficial to those with a tendency towards heat.

Advice for Qi and Blood Stagnation types

In Days 1–5 of your cycle, Qi Stagnant types need to put some time aside for quiet reflection. Because this tends to be an emotively driven condition, I think this is also good time to practise forgiveness.

To alleviate problems associated with Qi and Blood

FOODS THAT BENEFIT THE QI

Beef	Ham	Rice
Cherries	Herring	Royal jelly – fresh if available
Chicken	Lentils	Sweet potatoes
Coconut	Liquorice	Shiitake mushrooms
Dates	Mackerel	Squash
Figs	Molasses	Tofu
Ginseng	Oats*	Yam
Grapes	Potatoes	

* Oats have a regulatory effect on hormones, notably sex and thyroid hormones.

Stagnation try:
- lavender oil for the bath (Qi Stagnation) or chamomile, cypress, geranium, lemon and rose oils (Blood Stagnation)
- teas: jasmine, fennel, chamomile, spearmint
- drinking warm water first thing in the morning, with a twist of lemon
- gentle exercise – practise yoga daily, plus gentle walks
- tai chi and qigong – these are particularly great for Stagnation
- carrot and coriander soup
- chicken soup (see page 50)
- eating lightly
- rest (for a 'dragging sensation' – this can mean your Qi is weak) or for a 'sinking feeling'.

Also, some Stagnant types do find some exercise beneficial. Play around and find what you are comfortable with – belly dancing, perhaps?

Store cupboard for Qi and Blood Stagnation
Keep the following in your store cupboard:

- Aubergine
- Basil
- Cabbage
- Caraway
- Cardamom
- Carrot
- Cayenne
- Chestnuts
- Clove
- Coriander
- Dill seed
- Garlic
- Gooseberries
- Marjoram
- Orange peel
- Pickles
- Pine nuts
- Plums
- Prunes
- Radish
- Root vegetables
- Squash
- Star anise
- Sweet rice
- Tangerine peel
- Turmeric

Gubbins (as named by Jani's children)

This is a throw-it-all together way to use up leftover chicken, beef, mackerel, ham or tofu. It is excellent hot or cold, and makes a good supper as well as a portable lunch to take to work. Add any combination of carrots, sweet potatoes, peas and any other vegetable of your choice.

1. Cook some rice in stock (1 cup rice to 2 cups water is standard proportion) with 1 star anise and 2 cardamom pods and ¼ teaspoon of turmeric. Bring the rice and liquid to the boil, stir, cover and turn to lowest setting to simmer for 20–25 minutes. Don't take the lid off during cooking. The rice is cooked when the surface is pitted with holes and the grains are 'standing up'.

2. While the rice is cooking, sauté an onion and some garlic, then add the vegetables with a little water and sauté until cooked. When the rice is finished, transfer into a mixing bowl and 'fluff' the rice. Add the meat, fish or tofu, fold in the cooked vegetables and garnish with chopped parsley or coriander, chopped spring onions and any nuts or seeds of your choice.

Is the mind on board?

Affirmations

Say these in the morning and evening (and any other time you feel like it):

*   'I am letting go of the old, and looking forward to another chance to get healthy.'
*   'I can move freely now and without pain.'
*   'I am rebalancing, I am feeling happier and healthier and I am looking to the future.'
*   'This is a fresh start. I am leaving behind the last cycle and moving forward with optimism and hope.'

Qigong

It's lovely to practise qigong outside in nature, but this may not always be practical, so anywhere calm and quiet will do. Try these exercises in the mornings when your energy is up and when exercising can be invigorating rather than depleting.

Drawing the Bow to Shoot the Vulture
This exercise is suitable for everyone:
- Step to the left and squat down.
- Bring your palms together in front of your chest, then pull your right hand towards your right nipple in a fist shape and extend the left hand, as if pulling a bow.
- Stare to your left at an imaginary target.
- Bring your left hand down and across your body and then up to the right shoulder while breathing in.
- Now pull the left fist back to the left nipple and extend the right hand to the right, staring at a target to the right while you breathe out.

Repeat twelve times in each direction.

Shaking the Spine
- **Part 1:** Stand with arms by your side and your palms facing the floor – fingers forward. Stand still and calm the mind. Rise up on to tiptoes and breathe out. Stay as high as you can for three seconds, then drop your heels to the floor. Repeat 24 times.
- **Part 2:** Stand with your hands on your waist but with your fingers pointing backwards. Rise on to your tiptoes, hold for three seconds and then let yourself drop down. Repeat 24 times.
- **Part 3:** Stand with your hands just below your breasts (as if cupping them) with the palms facing the ceiling. Rise on to your tiptoes, hold for three seconds, then let yourself drop down. Repeat 24 times.

Yoga

Some yoga stretches are best practised in the morning in a calm, quiet environment – I would even recommend getting up a bit earlier to steal this time for yourself. It is really worth making time for this.

My colleague, yoga practitioner Uma Dinsmore-Tuli, also recommends poses for the evening (the moon sequence, for example) which are particularly helpful during menstruation. I have included a section on yoga for fertility in the Appendix (see pages 334–351). This section also includes advice on yoga during menstruation.

Note: do not 'invert' – e.g. do a headstand – when you have your period.

Recommendations for yoga during menstruation

There are some sequences and positions I particularly recommend during this phase:

1. Shakti bandha (freeing of feminine energy) *(three to five minutes)*. The 'Grinding the Mill' pose is particularly good (see page 338).

2. Chandra sequence (honouring the moon) *(five to nine minutes)* – these poses are best done in the evening (see page 340). When you have completed the honouring the moon sequence, move to hare pose. The hare pose and the hare-cobra pose (page 342) are very comforting for period pain.

It is a good idea to have a folded blanket or cushion under the knees throughout this practice. All the movements are done as you exhale.

Poses that are good for painful cramps

1. Hare pose (as described above).

2. Try resting on your back and hugging your knees into your chest. As you breathe out, draw the thighs in close to your belly *(apanasana)*.

3. Supportive forward bends can also provide comfort and relief: sit on the floor with your legs out straight. Put a bolster between the legs and rest forwards over it as a support. Use cushions or blocks to raise the height of your support until you can easily rest your forehead on it without straining your back. If you prefer a higher support, then have a chair between your legs with a cushion or bolster on the seat to provide support for your forehead as you rest forwards.

4. Some women prefer backward bending to relieve painful menstrual cramps, so experiment and find what works for you. The Camel pose (for instructions see the pre-ovulatory section in Chapter Five page 193) and the snake pose are both backward bends that relieve pain, but it's worth using them throughout the rest of the cycle to prevent or lessen future suffering during your period. So if you have regular period pains, do these as part of your daily routine.

5. Snake pose – this is a version of the cobra pose that many women find helpful during their period. Lie flat on your front with your forehead on the floor and your arms by your sides. Have your legs straight, your heels together. Bring your arms behind your back, moving your elbows as close together as you can. Place the palms together and interlock the fingers. Roll your shoulders down and back away from your ears, squeezing your shoulder blades together. Exhale. As you inhale, lift your head and raise the front of your chest up away from the floor. Exhale. Slowly lower the arms back down onto the back, tuck in the chin and gently rest the forehead on the floor. Move freely with the breath, up as you inhale and down as you exhale. If the pose suits you at this time, remain in the chest-lifted position for up to seven breaths. Keep your neck long and your shoulders well away from your ears. Feel your belly moving against the floor as you breathe fully.

Breathing techniques

If you are in need of balance and comfort during your bleeding time, you may enjoy a resting version of the seated alternate nostril practice that I also prescribe for the pre-menstrual phase. This can be done lying down at the start or end of your yoga programme; it has the same effect as alternate-nostril breathing, but with no hands.

This is a calming and quiet breath to balance the flow in the nostrils. It promotes tranquillity and ease. Allow your breath to come in through the right nostril. At the end of the inhalation, switch nostrils and allow the breath to leave through the left nostril. At the end of the exhalation, imagine your right nostril is closed and draw the next inhalation through the left nostril. At the end of that inhalation, switch nostrils and allow the breath to leave through the right nostril. This is one complete round. Do ten rounds in all.

Meditation

Inner silence, or meditation, is a powerful way to settle and can be especially helpful during menstruation. It can teach us to observe and understand the patterns of our own thoughts and emotions. You can practise it on its own or at the end of your yoga session.

Sit or lie comfortably in any pose that feels absolutely relaxed. Close your eyes and establish a full yogic breath (see Appendix for more on breathing).

EPSOM SALT BATH

Adding Epsom salts to your bath is a great way to relieve many menstrual discomforts. I also suggest it to women who suffer from fibroids. Epsom salts are beneficial because of their high magnesium sulphate content, which is absorbed through the skin as you soak.

- Put four cups of Epsom salts into your bath water
- Soak for twenty minutes
- Try to lie down and rest for fifteen minutes following your bath
- Use this time to do your affirmations.

1. **Listen** Listen to all the sounds around you. Start by bringing your attention to the loudest sounds first. Then, gradually, draw the focus of your awareness in closer until you listen to the quietest, closest sounds. Be aware of the sound of your own breath as it comes in and goes out.

2. **Touch** Shift the focus of your attention to the sense of touch. Become aware of the sensation of the breath passing into and out of the nostrils. Feel the cooler air coming in and the warmer air going out. Be aware of all the different textures and temperatures, which you can detect through touch. Feel if there is any difference between what you can feel on covered and uncovered skin. Then return to feeling the passage of air in the nose.

3. **Smell** Shift your attention and concentrate on any odours and aromas around you. Give your full attention to your sense of smell.

4. **Taste** Shift your attention to the sense of taste. Be aware of your tongue inside your mouth. Notice if there are sweet tastes, salty tastes, bitter, hot or astringent tastes. Give the sense of taste your full attention.

5. **See** Shift your attention to the sense of sight. Look into closed eyelids and be aware of whatever you may see there. Are there colours or shapes? Are there patterns or movement? Is it all blackness? Whatever there is to see, give your full attention to the sense of sight.

6. **Listen** Finally, return your attention to the sense of hearing, and become aware of the intimate sound of your own breath. Allow that breath to get a little louder, and use the sound of it as a bridge back over to awareness of other sounds in the room. Then widen your awareness until you are aware of sounds out in the wider world. When you are ready open your eyes.

Chapter Five

Days 6–13: Post-menstruation, Pre-ovulation

In this chapter, we will look at how to optimize the post-period, pre-ovulation phase. This is a hugely important and exciting part of the cycle; it is the week when you often feel most naturally creative, productive and positive.

Inside, the reproductive system is continuing its highly synchronized dance. The follicles are swelling, producing increasing levels of oestrogen, while the ripening egg is preparing to burst forth into the Fallopian tubes. In the womb, the first layers of the endometrium are being laid. The body is making preparations, and so must you.

In the clinic, I concentrate heavily on building Blood in this week. In China, many women drink a blood-recovering post-menstrual soup packed with Chinese herbs to nourish the blood. I have reproduced my own version, a watercress and spinach soup, on page 187.

Another area we want to optimize is the quality of your cervical mucus, which is essential for ensuring the smooth passage of sperm to egg, and egg to uterus.

Try to stay balanced in your emotions and practise your yoga sequences as often as you can.

Is the engine working?

Some women's cycles are as short as twenty-one days, while others go on for far longer than thirty-two days. In these cases, we need to look at what might be upsetting the cycle and how to rebalance it. This is a good time to rebalance an irregular cycle.

If you have an extended 'Yin phase' (i.e. this part of your menstrual cycle is over a week long), you may be Kidney Yin deficient, Damp or Qi Stagnant. For those of you who have very short cycles, this is the area you may have to work on, as you could be experiencing too much Heat.

How can you regulate your cycle?

The menstrual phase and this post-menstrual phase are usually the two times at which irregularities in the cycle manifest, so if you are experiencing either a long or a short cycle, it's worth concentrating some effort on this week.

Long follicular phase

This is when the egg is released too late in the follicular stage. In some women, it takes longer for the follicle to mature and the knock-on effect is that the whole cycle is slightly longer. Sometimes, this is because the woman is deficient in Blood and yin, which is why it is important to consider this aspect leading up to ovulation. Sometimes, the egg is mature, but does not release on time due to stagnation, usually caused by emotional tension and anxiety. Although the ultimate release of the egg will happen at the end of this phase, it is important that the issues are addressed prior to that time.

So, if you fit the description of a 'stagnant type', try to relax and enjoy yourself. Make use of your energy: you are often at your best at this stage of the cycle. Don't get hung up on ovulation; train your focus somewhere else – perhaps

BALANCING YIN AND YANG

As you know, Chinese medicine views the body in terms of energies – such as Qi, Yin and Yang – and prescribes a variety of treatments that seek to rebalance them. An imbalance of one of these energies can cause a blockage in the way that the body functions, and that can cause illness.

Yin is the cooling, moist and nourishing aspect of the body – it is like a soothing balm or nourishing fluid that runs through it. You need Yin to moisten your skin, your joints and to keep you generally lubricated. You also need it to keep your mind and emotions calm – without it you become restless, anxious and unable to 'switch off'. In fertility, Yin helps both men and women produce the secretions that are necessary for reproduction: plentiful Yin means plentiful cervical mucus and semen. A Yin Deficiency means a lower production of mucus and sperm.

Yang is the activating force in the body. It is 'warm' in essence and in the menstrual cycle it relates to the luteal (or incubator) phase (see Chapter Seven), when the egg is implanting. When Yang is deficient, the natural mechanisms of reproduction are slowed, the transportation of fluids is inhibited and you see the pooling of fluid. You slow down and begin to feel lethargic and lacking in 'get up and go'. A side effect may be a frequent need to urinate and difficulty in losing excess weight. Thought processes can also be sluggish, as can translating thought into action.

In Chinese medicine these energies – Qi, Yin and Yang – are essential to reproduction. Yin and Yang play out a balancing act throughout the cycle: Yin is dominant in the first phase, with Yang taking over after ovulation. The other thing to note is that in Chinese medicine, all the aspects of female reproduction are explained in terms of Kidney function, Heart function and the Womb.

The relationship between the Heart and the Womb is of particular importance in Chinese medicine, hence the phrase, 'bleeding Heart, bleeding Womb'. It's interesting how often this bond proves to be central in a diagnosis; I have unearthed an issue with the heart that has subsequently affected the womb in countless cases (see Electrocution case study, page 207).

These organs can possess their own Yin and Yang – or be deficient in the energies. Kidney Yin plays a crucial role in fertility. Someone who is 'Kidney Yin Deficient', for example, may experience night sweats and have a generally 'dry' appearance – their hair or skin will be dry and they may have a lack of body fluids, including cervical secretions. Those with Kidney Yin Deficiency are more prone to fertility issues.

Those with Kidney Yang Deficiency have a general lack of transforming energy which also means there is a tendency towards Coldness. Those who find it difficult to lose excess weight are often 'Yang Deficient' types.

on visualizations or yoga practice. This is the phase when you should have your free-spirit hat on – enjoy the idea that life is for living and being expansive.

Blood and Yin Deficient types will need to focus on preserving energy and cultivating good cervical mucus (which is not quite so much fun, I know), although I have tried to make it enjoyable for you with some suggestions below. (For more on cervical mucus see pages 94–5.)

Short follicular phase
This is when the egg is released too early, which has the knock-on effect of a short menstrual cycle, with the period coming early between Days 21 and 24. Sometimes, follicles are recruited and reach maturity too quickly, resulting in an egg that is not yet mature. It can happen as a woman reaches her menopause, but this is not the only cause; it can also happen when the hormones are out of balance – the egg may well be fertilized but not be viable. In Chinese medicine, this relates to too much Heat, usually generated because the Yin is deficient. Make sure that you follow my Heat-removing plan (see page 168) and introduce Yin (cool) nourishing foods and activities.

This may also happen when you are not ovulating. I recommend that you visualize the menstrual cycle with a strong emphasis on this phase (the bulging follicle and ripened egg) and on ovulation in the next chapter.

Recommendations
For everyone:
- Nourish your blood: see the section on diet below.
- Keep calm – practise meditation.
- Express your creative side – wear your 'free-spirit' hat occasionally.
- If you feel like being productive go for it, but don't wear yourself out.

- Drink nettle tea and raspberry leaf tea.
- Use essential oils – rose and geranium.
- Visualize the process – you can mentally correct irregularities in this phase.
- Stretch – the yoga sequence for this phase is my favourite.
- Make sex a priority at this stage! It's better to start early.

In addition the following can dry out your body's natural fluids, so avoid:
- medication for hay fever (antihistamines) – it dries fertile mucus
- alcohol
- tobacco
- caffeine
- air conditioning
- anywhere that is overheated
- too much time at the computer
- spicy foods.

Sex

I am going to start by prescribing sex whenever you feel like it. As I work in four-month cycles, emphasizing getting healthy before getting pregnant, I'm going to ask you to put the idea of conception to one side for a moment, and help you learn about your body and how it works. Fertility and conception are not the same thing.

So, take a break from focusing on conceiving and start enjoying sex for the sake of it – it's good for you. Some patients who have been trying to have a baby for a long time say that sex becomes a monthly chore, laden with baggage, pressure and, eventually, negative feelings. It becomes just another thing on a to-do list. But it's important to keep hold of the joy and the love. I often tell my patients that sex is like holidays;

the more you have, the more you want. And the more you want it, the more you enjoy it. And, as so many of us know, it's easy to lose sight of the joy of planning for a baby when conception doesn't happen straight away.

For those of you who *are* trying to conceive in this cycle, you can have sex with abandon this week as it's important that the sperm is already inside your reproductive tract prior to the release of an egg. I emphasize 'abandon' because I want you to have that sense of freedom and fun.

Q&A
How long should we have been trying before my partner (male) gets tested?
If a couple have been trying for a year (sooner in those over thirty-five) and there is no natural conception, then I advise that both partners be tested.

I urge you to think of your 'fertile time' as a period of up to five days, as your cycle can vary by a couple of days from month to month and sperm can sometimes live for up to four or five days in the Fallopian tube. One of my patients, for example, had her coil removed five days after she'd had sex and she fell pregnant that cycle. Another had sex on Day 9 of a usually regular twenty-eight-day cycle because she was trying to *avoid* her fertile time while on my four-month plan. She also fell pregnant. She told me: 'I had always been told that sperm could only live for seventy-two hours, but my sonographer [the person performing the scan] told me that medical science was revising that view and that he himself was pretty sure some sperm could live longer.'

Massage for your partner
I am a great believer in the power of the natural smell of our partners in sexual attraction and increasing libido. I also think massage has a very valuable role in making sex a more sensual and, therefore, more relaxed and pleasurable experience (there is nothing worse than trying to have sex when you are tense and tired). Don't be afraid of massage and don't try too hard – just relax.

Sandalwood is a wonderful essential oil that helps build libido in men – it has an exotic, heady smell and can really transport your mind away from a mundane day. Use one drop of essential oil for each millilitre of your base oil (a lot of people like almond oil, but you can use any base). A teaspoon of the combined mixture is usually enough for a massage.

Warm your hands by rubbing them together vigorously, then pour a small amount of oil on them and rub together again. Start by rubbing the oil on to your partner's tummy, moving in circular movements in a clockwise direction. Start with small circular movements around the navel and gradually increase the size of the circle as you continue outwards. Be careful to avoid the genitals as the oil can interfere with the sperm passage.

Rubbing the lower back over the kidney area, over the sacrum in large circular movements, is also very good for male sexual function.

Is the fuel good?

I asked a few colleagues what we could recommend to optimize this stage and they suggested a raspberry jelly and foods made with egg whites – including an egg white omelette.

Now, I realize that in this context, jelly may not sound that enticing, but in the wonderful world of Chinese medicine, we match like for like. If you can't face jelly, don't worry, but if you can, and it makes you laugh to recognize the symbolism, all the better. A sense of humour goes a long way in this process, and it certainly promotes wellbeing.

Other foods that can help are aloe vera, which you can take as a supplement, as well as royal jelly, honey, sesame seeds, seaweeds and all oily fish.

Store cupboard for all

As a general rule, when you are building Blood, think of black and dark green foods. Eating red meat is an easy way to build Blood, but it's not suitable for everyone. The following foods will help all types maximize this phase, so include them in your diet alongside any recommendations I made in the last chapter. If any of them are on your 'avoid' list, however, you should still do so; for example, Cold types still need to avoid watermelon and Damp types should avoid pork and duck.

- Apples
- Asparagus
- Avocados
- Amaranth flakes
- Beetroot
- Black beans
- Black sesame seeds
- Blackcurrants
- Carrots
- Cherries
- Dates
- Duck
- Eggs
- Honey
- Meat
- Nettle
- Oats
- Pear
- Pomegranate
- Pork
- Royal jelly – fresh, if you can find it
- Seaweed
- Dark leafy greens
- Sesame seeds
- Sweet potato
- Tofu
- Watermelon
- Yam

Raspberry Jelly

Serves 4
5 leaves gelatine
500g frozen raspberries
150g caster sugar
115g fresh raspberries

1. Soak the gelatine in cold water until it has softened. Meanwhile, put the frozen raspberries, sugar and 400ml water in a pan. Heat until the sugar has dissolved, then simmer for a couple of minutes.

2. Push the mixture through a sieve into a clean pan, return to the heat and add the gelatine (squeezing out any excess water), stirring until it has completely dissolved.

3. Strain into a jug and leave to cool.

4. Leave the mixture until it has started to thicken, then stir in the fresh raspberries and pour into a 1-litre mould.

5. Chill until just set (about 4 hours).

Mint Jelly

Serves 2
3½ leaves gelatine
large bunch mint leaves
200g caster sugar
juice of 3 limes

1. Soak the gelatine in cold water until it has softened and squeeze out excess water.

2. Pour the caster sugar into a pan with 200ml water; heat gently until it has dissolved, then simmer for a couple of minutes. Add the mint and leave to infuse for 10 minutes.

3. Strain into a clean pan and add the gelatine, heating the mixture until it has dissolved.

4. Add the lime juice, then strain into a jug and leave to cool until set.

Egg White Omelette

Serves 1
3 large egg whites
1 teaspoon water
pinch of ground pepper
1 teaspoon of vegetable oil

You can add whatever you like to the basic recipe, but as we are trying to boost Blood this week, I'd suggest spinach and possibly some goat's cheese.

1. Whisk the egg whites, water and pepper together in a mixing bowl until you achieve 'soft peaks'.

2. If you are using spinach and goat's cheese toss them together in a separate bowl.

3. Heat the frying pan with a teaspoon of oil. Pour in the mixture, coating the bottom of the pan, and cook over a medium heat until it starts to set.

4. Sprinkle on the spinach and goat's cheese, if using.

5. Fold half the omelette on to itself and cook for around a further 2 minutes.

Watercress & Spinach Soup

Serves 4

dash of olive oil

300g fresh spinach, washed

100g fresh watercress, washed

1 medium potato, diced

1 medium onion, chopped

850ml homemade chicken stock
(see page 50)

milk or water

½ tsp grated nutmeg

salt and pepper

1. Sauté the chopped onion in the olive oil until soft. Add the diced potato and after 3 minutes add the stock and simmer for a further 20 minutes, or until the potato is cooked.

2. Add the spinach leaves and cook on a slightly higher heat for about 5 minutes, stirring all the time to make sure all the leaves have wilted. Add the watercress.

3. Using a food processor or blender, liquidize the soup. Add a splash of milk or water if it is too thick and season with salt, pepper and nutmeg.

Chicken & Broccoli Risotto

Serves 5

1.2 litres (approx.) homemade chicken stock (see page 50)

1 tbsp olive oil

2 medium onions, chopped

2 cloves garlic, chopped

400g Arborio risotto rice

250g broccoli florets, divided into small, bite-sized pieces

4 cooked chicken breasts or meat from a small whole-roasted chicken, 'pulled' apart into small chunks

3 large handfuls chopped parsley

100g freshly grated Parmesan cheese

Maldon sea salt and black pepper

1. Warm the stock in a saucepan. In the meantime, put the oil in another large, heavy-bottomed pan and add the chopped onion. Cook over a medium heat with the lid on, stirring occasionally, for about 4 minutes.

2. Add the chopped garlic and cook for a further minute before adding the rice. Over a slightly higher heat, start to cook the rice, stirring continuously – you don't want it to stick to the pan or turn brown. Continue cooking the rice like this for about 4 minutes.

3. Turn down the heat to a low simmer and gradually start adding the stock, a little at a time, allowing it to be absorbed into the rice before the next addition. This process should take about 15–20 minutes in all. After about 10 minutes, add the broccoli florets and some salt and pepper. When the rice is nearly cooked, add the chicken pieces, chopped parsley and Parmesan. You may need to add a little more water if the risotto is sticking to the pan. Season to taste before serving.

For Cold

- Use the womb warmer (see page 81) every other day before ovulation if your tummy is cold to touch below the navel.
- Use abdominal massage every day leading up to ovulation.
- Stick to warm foods in the diet.
- Keep your bedtime routine cosy: a bath with oils, warm bed, hot-water bottle.
- Use essential oils to warm: jasmine (also a fantastic aphrodisiac), cedarwood, basil.
- Exercise is good for Cold types in this phase.
- Try some emotional warmth, such as catching up with friends and family.
- Perhaps you could watch some heart-warming films?

For Damp

I always feel conscious that Damp draws a bit of short straw when it comes to diet, but you can make up for it by enjoying other areas of your life, such as getting out for nice walks and moving around to get things flowing. Try yoga or pilates, for example.

- Stay vigilant about the diet (you don't want your secretions to be too thick).
- Keep your food light and steer clear of any junk.
- Remember that too much fluid in the run-up to ovulation can interrupt the sperm's journey to the egg and the egg's passage down the Fallopian tube.
- Use abdominal massage every day until ovulation.
- Enjoy exercising.
- Enjoy plenty of sex if you feel like it.

For Blood Deficient

It almost goes without saying that during this phase, when building Blood is of vital importance, Blood Deficient patients really have to take extra-good care of themselves.

- Again: lots of rest and early nights.
- An incredibly nourishing diet will really help.
- Attempt a little exercise now, but nothing too depleting.

For Heat

As you approach ovulation, you need to pay attention to any changes in your secretions – do they resemble egg whites? If you have no secretions, or they are very scant, you need to concentrate on cooling and relaxing.

- Try cool, wet visualizations – perhaps a gentle waterfall?
- Stick to cooling foods (see recipe for mint jelly on page 186).
- When you meditate, imagine your skin plumping up.
- Try essential oils: chamomile, cypress, geranium, lemon and rose – again, dilute them for massage with a carrier oil, such as almond, or use a few drops neat in the bath.
- You could also benefit from putting your 'free-spirit' hat on – let go and relax!
- Stay hydrated, but remember to sip your water, don't gulp.
- If you can, book a session with the acupuncturist or herbalist.

There's a recipe for raspberry jelly on page 186, but if you are very overheated try the one for mint jelly instead.

For Qi Stagnation

Patients with Qi stagnation need exercise in this phase, so a good walk every morning would be good or swimming if you enjoy it. Otherwise, try Qigong or yoga. You could also:

- Use essential oils: grapefruit, lavender, mandarin and bergamot – either diluted for massage, or neat in the bathwater.
- Get talking – phone friends to chat.
- Get things off your chest – in a positive way (no arguing!).
- Make plans – do you have some ideas to throw about?
- Feel grateful – think about keeping a gratitude diary. Try to put something in it every day this week.

For Blood Stagnation

If you carry on with dark spotting after your period it's likely that your Blood Stagnant problem is still present. If it doesn't improve with this programme alone, you'll need to think about acupuncture or get a referral to a gynaecologist to check for endometriosis.

- Use essential oils: chamomile, cypress, geranium, lemon and rose.
- I recommend exercise; belly dancing, in particular, is so appropriate for those with Blood Stagnation.
- Use abdominal massage every day until ovulation.

Is the mind on board?

On the wall of my treatment room is a beautiful painting which was given to me by a patient. She painted it when she conceived her third child after a long period of trying. This patient had spent five years bringing up her first two children and had to some degree neglected her own needs. Of course she was delighted to be a mother but felt she had lost touch with her creativity. I urged her to stop focusing on trying for the third baby for a while and to take up something creative that would give her joy in another way. I explained how important the part of the menstrual cycle is which leads up to ovulation and how instead of thinking about creating a baby she could try to take her mind off it by creating something else. This amazing woman used this time to create both the beautiful painting which now hangs on my wall and, in due course, the beautiful daughter which completed her family.

The lesson to learn is that sometimes these fertile activities nourish us on an emotional level and allow us to be creative, literally making us more fertile. The follicular phase is an especially powerful time to start new and creative projects.

Affirmations

I recommend that you say your affirmations every morning and every night, but try to squeeze them in whenever you can beyond that. For example, when you are out taking a stroll, riding your bike, in the car, in the loo, or in the bath and any time other time you are alone and able to focus on them.

- 'I produce healthy fluids which nourish and grow my follicles to full maturity.'
- 'My body is filled with nourishing and cooling fluids that moisten my Fallopian tubes and smooth the passage of my egg.'
- 'I enjoy loving, sensual activities with my partner and we make love because we desire each other.'
- 'I put time aside to enjoy being with my partner for the sake of spending time together and enjoying each other's company.'
- 'My body produces thick, healthy blood in plentiful amounts to nourish my follicles and thicken my endometrium.'
- 'I am relaxed, happy and enjoy doing the things that make me feel fulfilled.'

Qigong
The Small Heavenly Cycle

Stand with your feet hip-width apart and knees slightly bent. Your fingertips should be directed in towards the lower belly below the navel. Sense the connection with the subtle energy system inside your lower belly.

Trace the Qi down the centre line of your abdomen in your mind, past the pubic bone and between your legs, through the genitalia and pelvic floor to the anus. Bring your hands around to the back of your pelvis to the sacrum and up the lumbar spine. Continue up the spine as far as you can between the shoulder blades. Continue to trace the Qi up your back and over the top of the centre of the head, then slowly and gently, coming down the centre line of the head, face, throat, chest, solar plexus, upper abdomen and back to the lower abdomen.

To close the practice, simply stand or sit with fingers directed into the lower abdomen and concentrate the Qi in that direction.

Traditionally, this loop is meditated upon as if two snakes are chasing each other. The one in front has a pearl in its mouth (the magic pearl of life) and the one behind is trying

QIGONG

Qigong is a Chinese practice which involves slow graceful movements and controlled breathing techniques; it is both a form of exercise and meditation. The aim of the practice is to promote the circulation of Qi in a similar way to acupuncture (without the needles) and by doing so it has a positive effect on both physical and emotional health. In the same way as with the yoga, I worked with my friend John Tindall to develop movements for each phase of the cycle to enhance the natural process.

to obtain it. I love this image. I think of the pearl as the egg that is about to be released at ovulation; it is very powerful for fertility.

Yoga

The focus for yoga practice here is to nourish and grow. Give full attention to your breath and use the description below to help you form a mental connection with your ovaries.

- Full yogic breath and inner awareness (five to ten minutes) – see page 336.
- Seed to flower: alternating between opening and protection (three to five minutes) – see page 337.
- Honouring the moon (*Chandra namaskara*) – see Appendix, page 340. This practice can be done in the evening.
- Focus your attention on that sense of growth and expansion: pay attention to the feeling of openness all the way down to your fingertips. Flex your fingers into the tips as you practise *Chandra namaskara*.

Camel pose (Ustrasana)

This pose can also feel good at this time of the cycle and it fits well within the moon sequence, just before the final forward bend.

1. Kneel with thighs vertical and knees hip-width apart. Have your toes tucked forwards and the balls of your feet on the floor. Place your palms on your buttocks, fingers pointing down.
2. Breathe into your abdomen and chest. Keep your spine extended, then slowly move your hands down the back of your thighs as far as is comfortable. Only go as far as you can while keeping the thighs vertical. Encourage the front of your chest forwards with a big inhalation, and keep your shoulders down, away from your ears. Only if

it feels easy for you to do so, move your hands lower at this point, then grasp your heels. Wherever your hands are, keep your thighs vertical insofar as you are able, so that your hips are directly above your knees as you draw your shoulder blades together behind you, moving them down towards your waist and opening your chest.

3. Keep your spine extended, so that your lower back is comfortable and long. Keep your chest and belly moving rhythmically with an easy breath.

4. Only if and when you feel balanced, with equal weight on your knees and hands, should you point your chin up to the ceiling, keeping the back of your neck long. If your chin points to the ceiling, don't drop the weight of your head back, and keep length in the neck.

CASE STUDY: THE POWER OF AFFIRMATION, AFFIRMED

A man came in to my clinic with his girlfriend. He was born and bred in Essex and worked for one of the top city banks. He seemed to be one of the least likely candidates for the Male Cycle I'd come across.

When I talked about affirmations he didn't look in the least bit fazed. I asked if he knew what I meant. 'I've been bigging myself up in the mirror every single morning since I did my "A" levels,' he said, without a hint of embarrassment. 'How do you think I got where I am today?' He then proceeded to tell me that his mother, a single parent with very little money, had brought up four children on morning affirmations and positive thinking. They'd all gone on to further education – he went to one of the top universities in the country – despite the fact that no one in their family had done so before. And all four went on to find high-flying jobs.

He took the Male Cycle completely in his stride and I was really proud of both partners when they came in together to tell me they had conceived.

5. Breathe for up to nine rounds of breath in the pose, but start out with just one or two, until you feel easy in this expansive backbend.

6. To release from the pose, slowly move your chin down and your hands back up your legs to your buttocks. On an inhalation, release your hands from behind your back and return to standing. On an exhalation, fold forwards into the hare pose and lengthen your spine. Breathe into your belly and feel it moving against your thighs. Rest forwards for as long as you held the camel pose.

Half-shoulder stand (vipariti karani)

This stage can also be a helpful time to use a therapeutic inversion:

1. Lie on your back, tucking your knees into your belly.

2. Using your hands to support your hips, let the weight of your legs and buttocks transfer down through your elbows into the floor. Once you feel comfortable, lift your knees up away from your belly and let your legs straighten, so that they are held upwards at an angle of about 45 degrees over your head. Breathe fully in the pose.

3. To come down, bend your knees into your belly and roll back to the floor.

Q&A

Can electrical currents from devices such as. mobile phones and laptops affect male fertility?
Yes, any source of heat can potentially damage sperm. This would include using a laptop directly on your lap. The evidence on mobile phone use showed that those who used the phone for more than four hours a day had a reduced sperm count.

How often should my sperm be tested?
It is often necessary to re-test following an abnormal result as one test alone can be misleading. Sperm is sensitive so even if the male partner has produced a child in the past or has had normal sperm results it does not mean his sperm will remain within normal range. It is especially worth testing after an illness, particularly an illness with a fever. I normally suggest twice and then every six months if there is no pregnancy.

THE THREE-MONTH MALE CYCLE

This cycle is suitable for men:
- who want to improve their health prior to conceiving
- who have had a poor semen analysis
- whose partner has had repeat miscarriages or failed IVF.

Read through Chapter Three (Your fertility type) – it all applies to you too (except the menstrual cycle section) and I have added a few more 'male' symptoms below. You will fall into one or more of the following broad categories:
- Hot man – Yin Deficient
- Stagnant man
- Cold man – Yang Deficient
- Damp (Damp/Heat) man

Men generally are not as good as women at thinking about their health, but I want you to reflect on how you feel. Ask yourself the following questions:
- How is your energy (out of ten)?
- When did you feel better than this?
- What has changed?
- How do you feel about sex these days? Are you experiencing any problems with desire or performance? (If so, you and your partner may need to sit down and talk about how you are feeling towards the baby-making plan or speak to a professional.)
- Are you spending a lot of time in the office to avoid facing other areas in your life that are not working so well?

- How is your diet?
- Are you drinking and smoking? How do you feel about these things and do you still need them in your life?

Just thinking about your health in a more focused way may highlight areas that need to be worked on. I am now going to ask you some questions relating directly to sex and performance which, when added to the information from Chapter Three, will help you to determine your type.

Are you a Cold man – Kidney Yang Deficient?

Just as women need a warm womb in order to conceive, men too need to have warmth in their body to produce active sperm. This idea is not so foreign to us: think of the saying 'fire in your belly'. Ask yourself – do you still have fire in your belly?
- Do you suffer from a lack of libido?
- Do you suffer from lower backache and general lower-back weakness?
- Do your genitals or lower abdomen feel cold to the touch?
- Do you suffer from slight incontinence?

Cold may result in low sperm count and poor motility (its ability to move). In clinic, I recommend acupuncture for these men around the time of their partner's ovulation to help with motility.

Are you a Hot man – Kidney Yin Deficient?

Too much heat is not a good thing for sperm either. We talked at length earlier about how heat can damage sperm. Do you have a good libido but are unable to sustain an erection?

- Do you sometimes get the beginnings of an erection but cannot maintain it?
- Is your ejaculate scanty?
- Do you feel restless?
- Do you feel agitated?
- A high number of abnormally formed spermed may mean the sperm can not penetrate the egg.

Are you a Stagnant man?

Stagnation usually manifests itself on an emotional level, but can then develop into a physical problem. See the section on stagnation on page 132. Some pointers are:

- Do you have pain and distension in your testicles?
- Do you suffer from lack of libido due to disinterest?
- Do you spend a lot of time sitting at a desk?
- Do you feel depressed and disconnected from sex and life in general?
- Do you feel dissatisfied with life?
- Do you sigh a lot?

Good movement of Qi and Blood is vital to propel the sperm from the testicles to the penis and to maintain an erection. This is well treated with acupuncture.

Are you a Damp (or Damp/Heat) Man?

As with women, the Damp condition is often linked to diet but can be caused by damp living conditions. It is always a factor in cases of infection and STDs.

- Do you suffer from flaccidity?
- Do you have a history of STDs?
- Do you have genital itching?
- Do your genitals feel hot and damp?
- Do you have any discharge from your penis?
- Does your ejaculate have a smell to it?
- Is your ejaculate slightly yellow in colour?
- Have you been told that your sperm is 'clumped'?

Recommendations

For everyone:

- Stop smoking.
- Don't smoke marijuana.
- Take charge of your sexual health – make sure you see your doctor if you suspect that you may have any STDs or low-grade infections.
- Limit your exposure to chemicals which are harmful to sperm (see page 46).
- If you are overweight you will need to lose some of the excess.
- Take exercise; it is good for your sperm. (But don't overexercise – see 'Iron Man', page 276.)

- Don't cycle; the pressure cycling places on the perineum during cycling can cause Stagnation.
- Don't go into steam rooms.
- Eat liquorice.
- Ginseng supplements improve the blood flow to the penis and may improve sexual function in some patients.
- Do pelvic-floor exercises.
- Follow the diet plan according to your type (see pages 158–171) and see 'Nutrition', below.

Acupuncture

Acupuncture is beneficial in raising general health and vitality levels in men. Extensive research has also shown acupuncture to be effective in improving sperm count, motility and morphology (the shape of the sperm cells). Furthermore, it has been used for thousands of years to treat all manner of male health issues, particularly in the area of fertility and reproduction. After an initial course of acupuncture, I often recommend that men receive more at the time of their partner's ovulation to improve sperm motility and sexual function.

Hypnotherapy, meridian tapping and visualization

These supporting therapies can be helpful to men as well as women wanting to improve their health prior to conception. Visualization and hypnotherapy are useful tools for stress management. Visualization has also been effective for helping patients who need to increase their sperm count. Men can also have unconscious underlying emotional blocks which may contribute to reduced fertility. These can be treated with meridian tapping (see page 321).

Some of these techniques are very effective for alcohol management and quitting smoking, both of which have a profound effect on fertility, as well as helping to boost confidence (see case study, below).

Nutrition

Nutrient depletion, smoking, alcohol intake and heavy metal toxicity (see page 46, for more on environmental factors) can all have a destructive influence on male fertility. So, good nutrition plays an important role here and is vital for healthy sperm.

Essential nutrients include the minerals selenium and zinc and vitamins C and E. The average British diet contains 30mcg selenium per day, while the recommended daily intake for men is 75mcg. It's a good idea to introduce some of the following foods into your diet:

- **For zinc:** oysters, pumpkin seeds, whole wheat, rye, oats, almonds and peas.
- **For selenium:** tuna, sesame seeds, shellfish, avocados and wholegrains.
- Other beneficial foods include oily fish, peppers, broccoli, cauliflower, cabbage, spinach, chicken and fish.

Chapter Six

Day 14: Ovulation

The miracle of the moment of conception is precisely that:
a miracle. Western medicine cannot, as yet, explain how
exactly the meeting of sperm and egg can fuse to create the
brand new single cell of a separate entity.

Through the extraordinary advances of Assisted Reproduction Techniques, we can now artificially perform the role
of nature. We cannot, however, guarantee that the sperm will
fertilize the egg, that a fertilized egg (blastocyst) will implant
or that an embryo will become a foetus and go all the way
to produce a healthy newborn baby thirty-eight or so weeks
later. There are no guarantees in either nature or science.

What we can do, however, is pool all the available information – from both Eastern and Western medicine – to create
the best and healthiest conditions for the miracle of conception to occur. Some parts of the process remain a mystery,
but it's worth arming ourselves with as much information as
possible before we start. When I first see a patient or patients,
I try to gauge how much they understand about the way their
bodies work and how conception occurs. It's not a test, but
many couples are amazed to discover how little they know.

Around 10 per cent of women come to me because they are not ovulating. If this is the case for you, I want you to follow the recommendations in this chapter while taking fifteen minutes out of your morning to visualize releasing an egg on Day 14. Keep following the recommendations while we work on getting you to ovulate.

Ovulation

It is official: we all like to get a little flirty, a little coquettish and a little mischievous around the time of ovulation. It's not totally our fault: that most feminine of hormones, oestrogen, comes in to play as we go out to play.

Research has shown that our faces, scent and voice all become more 'attractive' when we reach our fertile period and our bodies increase oestrogen production in order to facilitate ovulation. We also become more confident, have more energy, a heightened sense of taste and smell and we are more

---

MULTIPLE OVULATION

Multiple ovulation occurs when more than one egg is released. The second egg will be released within 24 hours of the first egg, but after that window no more eggs will be released in that cycle. If both eggs are fertilized and then implant, non-identical twins have been conceived.

It's thought that as we get older our bodies are more likely to release more than one egg, making mothers over 35 more likely to conceive twins naturally (1 in every 80 births is naturally conceived twins). However, doctors now believe that multiple ovulation may occur much more frequently – in as many as 5 to 10 per cent of all cycles – but that the second foetus frequently miscarries. This is known as the 'vanishing twin phenomenon'.[1]

interested in having sex.

Hormones underpin your cycle, and understanding just how they keep it turning is key to getting to grips with the way you feel at different times. Outside influences, such as alcohol and drugs, can tamper with your hormonal balance and make the natural changes in your cycle much more challenging. It is easier to cope with some of the ups and downs of your hormones if your life is balanced and healthy.

OVULATION: THE EGG RELEASES FROM THE FOLLICLE

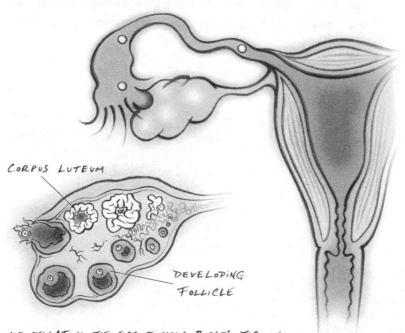

CORPUS LUTEUM

DEVELOPING FOLLICLE

AT OVULATION THE EGG FINALLY BURSTS THROUGH, OR RUPTURES, THE FOLLICLE AND IS RELEASED INTO THE OVARY FROM WHERE IT CONTINUES ITS JOURNEY ALONG THE FALLOPIAN TUBE. IF THE EGG MEETS A SPERM TO FERTILIZE IT THIS IS THE BEGINNING OF A NEW LIFE.

How ovulation works

On Days 12 and 13, FSH and oestrogen levels rise high enough for the process of ovulation to begin. The pituitary gland releases more LH which stimulates one (occasionally more) ripened egg to rise to the surface of the follicle.

On Day 14, the egg (or eggs) bursts through the protective follicle, propelled by the release of prostaglandins, and is released into the adjacent Fallopian tube. This is ovulation.

In the days following ovulation, progesterone surges and you enter the luteal phase (described in the next chapter). In Chinese medicine, this is where Yin energy peaks and then the energy switches to Yang. Yin energy shares the qualities of oestrogen, while Yang shares the qualities of progesterone.

Is the engine working?

When everything is in good working order, you have a 30 per cent chance of conceiving at this point in the month. Ovulation is generally on Day 14; as I said in the last chapter, however, you should aim to have slightly more sex than normal from Day 10 if you are trying to conceive.

To work out when you are ovulating, look for changes in your cervical mucus (see page 94) along with, perhaps, a twinge in your ovaries. You may also experience tenderness in your breasts or nipples, abdominal bloating and heightened sensitivity. Those who are charting will be able to read ovulation in a rise in temperature.

Recommendations for everyone

What you need at ovulation is a really good flow of Qi. Any tension or anxiety might impede or prevent the release of an

Q&A

Do I ovulate from alternating ovaries? **This is normal female physiology, but each of us has our own unique pattern and although this is 'the norm' it is by no means the only way it occurs.**

egg, so the emphasis is on staying relaxed and happy, which is what should come naturally at this point in the cycle.

Once you start paying attention to your cycle, you may notice a change in your mood. Most women feel more carefree and open at this point. Scientists say you are more likely to 'notice' men around you, and you may find your inner flirt. It can be quite disconcerting to recognize just how much your hormones control your temperament and behaviour, but they are on your side. So, go with the flow!

Q&A

Can sexual positions determine whether you are more likely to conceive a girl or boy?
Sexual positions have no influence. The X chromosome containing sperm are generally heavier and more slow moving than the Y chromosome.

Things to do during the ovulation phase

- Concentrate on building Qi.
- Use meditation to avoid getting stressed.
- Try essential oils: lavender, rose, ylang ylang, neroli and melissa. Use them neat in the bath or diluted in a carrier oil for massage. These all help the heart–womb connection and bring about feelings of wholeness – that connection within.
- Drink tea: chamomile is calming and will help you to stay balanced at this exciting time.
- Try abdominal massage to invigorate Qi and blood in the abdomen.
- Increase your intake of essential fatty acids.
- Use the power of visualization (see case study, page 207).

In addition, there are some things to beware of

- Don't flood your system with water.
- Don't be tempted to take cough mixture to thin your mucus – you need to work on your fluids.
- Don't use lubricants or saliva as a lubricant.

Emma's Butternut Squash & Chestnut Risotto

Because the flow of Qi is very important here, I thought I'd give you my own favourite Qi-building recipe. Chestnuts are warming and good for yang and Qi. Butternut squash is also good for the Qi and cumin and thyme are warming for Cold types.

Serves 5

knob of butter
4 medium leeks, trimmed and sliced
1 tsp ground cumin
2 cloves garlic, chopped
900g butternut squash, peeled, deseeded and cubed
375 g Arborio risotto rice
1 litre hot vegetable stock (or chicken stock for Blood Deficient types)
1 tsp fresh thyme sprigs
250g chestnuts (either tinned, vacuum-packed or as nature intended)
salt and pepper
fresh Parmesan shavings

1. Gently heat the butter in a saucepan and cook the leeks, cumin, garlic and squash for 8 minutes, stirring occasionally; they need to be soft but not browned.

2. Stir in the rice until it is coated, then turn down the heat and add the stock, a ladle at a time. All the liquid must be absorbed before adding more. Add half the thyme and the chestnuts (broken into smaller pieces) with the last addition of liquid.

3. Season with salt and pepper and serve with Parmesan shavings.

Chai

Serves 2 in cups, 1 in a mug

350ml water
2 tsp sugar
½ stick cinnamon
½ tsp honey
8 cardamom pods
3 tsp Darjeeling tea leaves
8 whole cloves
5mm fresh ginger root, thinly sliced
150ml milk (or, for a chai latte, 120ml plus frothed milk at the end)

1. Pour the water into a saucepan over a medium/high heat. Add the cinnamon, cardamom, cloves and ginger and bring to the boil.

2. Lower the heat and simmer for 10 minutes with the lid on.

3. Add the milk, honey and sugar and continue to simmer; don't boil.

4. Remove from the heat, add the tea leaves and allow to steep for two to three minutes.

The moment of ovulation

As I've said before, the Heart has an important role in ovulation (remember the link between Heart and Womb in Chinese medicine), and if it is experiencing emotional tension or anxiety, whether from a recent or a more deep-rooted cause, this can impact on ovulation.

Some women can actually feel themselves ovulate; they say it is similar to a dull ache or a twinge on one side. This is reassuring, even encouraging, as it shows they are aware of their bodies and what is happening. However, I am always worried if someone reports feeling actual pain as they ovulate, as pain is not a normal aspect of this process. If a patient reports pain during ovulation to me, I will usually treat them for emotional issues as well and try to get to the root of any tension or anxiety.

Having said that, it is estimated that as many as 20 per cent of women do experience some pain or discomfort at the point of ovulation. In Western medicine this is termed 'mittelschmerz', which literally, translated from the German, means middle pain. The pain lasts for a couple of hours in most women, but in extreme cases is said to last a couple of days. Other symptoms can be 'light spotting' (a tiny amount of blood), nausea and cramps. Some of the advice given to relieve mittelschmerz is very similar to that in Chinese medicine – warming pads (a hot-water bottle or a bath) and rest.

Q&A

Do I ovulate every month? Most women will ovulate every month, but this is not guaranteed. If you have a regular menstrual cycle it is likely that you are ovulating and simple tests such as the ovulation test sticks (see page 206) may help identify when ovulation has occurred. Some women find it helpful to use these sticks along with measuring their temperature.

Not ovulating?

If you are not ovulating regularly (often this is the case in women with PCOS), I would use acupuncture points on the abdomen and over the ovaries, attached to an electro acupuncture machine, which is also attached to points on the ankle that relate to the reproductive system. (See Chapter 8.) This treatment has proved to be very helpful in Blood Stagnant or Damp types, who find it difficult to release an egg. However, in Blood Deficient types this is not a good treatment.

The case study below also shows just how fantastic it can be to visualize the image of the egg releasing. It is also essential reading for those who want to understand the relationship between Heart and Womb in Chinese medicine.

OVULATION TEST STICKS

Ovulation sticks measure the levels of luteinizing hormone (LH) in the urine. When there is a 'surge' this indicates the egg is about to be released. This is the optimum time for sex, but before and after this surge is also recommended to increase your chances.

Digital reading sticks seem to be the easiest to use and the most accurate, so it is worth spending the extra money on these as it reduces any doubt.

Pros

Ovulation sticks can be helpful if you:

- have an irregular cycle who don't know when they are ovulating
- don't experience any physical changes at this time, i.e. cervical mucus
- spend time away from their partners because of work commitments and cannot guarantee regular sex throughout the cycle
- are wondering if they are ovulating at all (if you find you are not, follow my advice).

Cons

- They can cause more and unnecessary distress for those who are worried about ovulation.
- Those couples who are tense around sex, may find they add to the pressure.
- Some women become too reliant on them and stop listening to their own bodies.
- They put too much focus on the time of ovulation, rather than sex and intimacy around the entire cycle.

CASE STUDY: SHE'S A BELIEVER

Some years ago, a woman in her early twenties came to me for treatment. Her symptom was that she had never had a natural bleed. Her gynaecologist prescribed Provera so that she would experience what is known as a 'break-away bleed', but he had also referred her to me. I knew I had a lot to prove as usually, someone this young would be sent down a different path.

I did the 360-degree diagnosis and, after much talking, I discovered that she had been electrocuted at the age of fourteen. I felt this was significant. I decided to treat the Heart Qi, which would have been damaged by the force of the shock.

She had other symptoms too: vivid dreams, panic attacks and a distracted, nervous demeanour, all of which were relevant.

I told her how I planned to proceed. I explained that I would need to recreate the natural rhythm of her menstrual cycle with acupuncture and that I would use the needles to recreate the energy of each phase. As she didn't actually have a cycle, we decided to make the first day of treatment her mid-cycle, so I stimulated the ovaries.

We agreed that the following week would be spent concentrating on the movement of Qi in the abdomen, mirroring the egg moving down the Fallopian tube. I told her that in the third week we could expect a bleed. As I described the treatment, I realized I was telling her the outcome as though it were an absolute given, while in my mind, I was slightly less confident. I had to stop myself from limiting my own expectations. I also treated her heart.

After the first treatment I gave her some reading material and explained that she had a big part to play. Her job was to go away and read what happens in the menstrual cycle and to visualize all of it happening in her own womb.

She duly came back for her second treatment and, after the third week she returned saying she had done exactly what I had asked. Then, somewhat matter-of-factly, she added: 'It worked as you said it would. The bleed came as I was leaving your clinic last week.'

I resisted the temptation to let my jaw hit the floor! Her cool nonchalance was incredible; she must have been totally unaware of the medical improbability of her situation. But I took away my own lesson here: my diagnosis was thorough and good and my treatment was effective; however, this young girl's role was crucial. Her mind was on board and her faith in her own ability was absolute.

It's my firm belief that treatment is most effective when the patient engages in the process and gives their mind to it – as this young girl did so brilliantly.

Is the fuel good?

From a Chinese medicine point of view, we are trying to encourage the movement of Qi and Blood in order to release an embryo.

For Cold
This is an interesting time for both Cold and Heat types because it symbolizes the crossover between the Yin and Yang phases of the cycle. Remember: Yin is cool and Yang is hot. In some ways you should achieve some natural balance here, which will only be enhanced if you have been following my recommendations.

So, until now you will have been concentrating on keeping your womb warm and no doubt your efforts will have had an effect. Around ovulation, I want you to draw on both the Yin and the Yang – the cooling elements, as well as the warming ones.

It's not very Chinese, I know, but I love prescribing chai for my Cold patients. You can make your own chai tea (see page 204) or, for a chai latte, just add frothed milk instead of warm milk. Another Indian dish that is great here is the korma curry (or any similar curry made with coconut milk) – the spices are warming, while the coconut milk is very cooling.

For Damp
This is a crucial phase of the cycle if you are a Damp type as you are likely to encounter problems releasing an egg if you are 'clogged up'. These are some of the things you need to keep in mind at this time:
• Remain calm and avoid stress.
• Your diet must be as clear as possible now – stick closely to my recommendations and avoid dairy, sugar, processed foods and wheat. But remember: it is as much about

introducing those foods that will help your type as it is about eliminating those that are bad for you.

- Book a massage – perhaps take along one of the oils suggested above?
- Visualize and meditate – you will find it very empowering at this stage.
- Remember the connection between the Heart and the Womb – think of the Qi flowing uninhibited.
- Practise the yoga for ovulation (see page 214) – really feel yourself open up and release.
- Acupuncture is very useful at ovulation particularly for Damp types.

For Blood deficient

Both Heat and Blood deficient types may experience some mid-cycle spotting or bleeding. If the blood is bright red, it's Heat. If it's pale and watery, it is more likely to be a sign of Blood deficiency.

While my advice to Blood deficient types is rest, rest, rest, until you have built up your Blood again, this might be the one phase in your cycle when you feel your heart bursting with energy. Don't overdo it though; you need to keep your energy reserves well stocked for the last phase of the cycle when building a healthy and plump womb lining will draw on all your resources.

PHLEGM

Patients who have had a tendency towards Damp for a long time can often experience phlegm. This is particularly pronounced in PCOS patients for whom everything becomes a little glue-like or sticky. Add some of the following foods to your diet:

- Almonds
- Apple peel
- Button mushrooms
- Garlic
- Grapefruit
- Lemon peel
- Liquorice
- Marjoram
- Mustard leaf
- Mustard seed
- Olives
- Onions
- Orange peel
- Pears
- Peppers
- Peppermint
- Persimmon
- Radishes
- Seaweed
- Shiitake mushrooms
- Shrimp
- Tea
- Thyme
- Walnuts
- Watercress

I recommend that you:

- eat green foods – such as dark green vegetables
- eat black foods – mulberry, liquorice and black mushrooms are all good
- don't over-exert your eyes – avoid long periods in front of the computer and take regular breaks[6]
- drink ginseng tea
- use essential oils
- watch some comedy – laughing boosts the immune system which is great for Blood deficient types, so go out and rent some *Seinfeld*, or whatever it is that tickles you
- get as close to eight hours' sleep as you can
- rest your mind – gentle meditation is good
- spend some time listening to your favourite music – this is a great distraction for Blood Deficient types.

For Heat

Let me reiterate what I said to those with Cold tendencies, above: the mid-cycle is the crossover between the Yin (cooling) and Yang (warming) phases of the cycle. Your Fallopian tubes need the requisite amount of fluid to move the egg into the womb and the endometrium (womb lining) needs to be plump and receptive for implantation. Be careful not to dry out.

It is especially important that you avoid caffeine and alcohol around this time as they are heating substances. Enjoy being natural and free – if you have Heat tendencies, you'll have enough energy during ovulation without any additional stimulants. Any bright red mid-cycle spotting is likely to be a sign of Heat. Recommendations for Heat types at ovulation include:

- fresh mint tea (steep fresh mint in hot water until it is cool enough to drink)
- white tea and green tea (with a hint of lemon, if preferred)

- foods that are blue (such as blueberries), purple or green
- a warm bath or shower – not hot
- using mint essential oil – either in the bath or diluted for massage
- cooling cucumber eye mask or the cucumber fool, right
- cooling exercise, such as swimming or yoga
- walking away from stressful situations or confrontations (one patient was so determined not to get het up that she stopped driving while she was trying to conceive because she knew this was the time she was most likely to lose her temper!)
- avoiding the temptation to take things personally
- meditation.

For Qi Stagnation

My advice to those who are Qi Stagnant is to:

- avoid sugar and stimulants (even though you will crave them)
- chew your food really well
- make an effort to be happy and relaxed while eating; make it an event
- avoid emotionally difficult subjects (which can impair the flow of Qi to the ovaries)
- visualize 'releasing' and 'letting go'.

Cucumber Fool

Serves 2

3 large cucumbers
white wine vinegar
pinch of salt
handful of watercress
3 spring onions, chopped
fresh dill
pinch of sugar
parsley
freshly ground white pepper
dollop of soured cream (optional)

1. Peel and halve the cucumbers lengthways, scraping out the seeds and juice (reserve the juice) and setting them to one side in a mixing bowl. Add the salt and allow them to drain.

2. Cut the cucumber halves into large chunks and set aside.

3. In a food processor, whiz the cucumber chunks with the spring onions and the sugar. Season with the pepper and few of drops of white wine vinegar (to taste).

4. Add the reserved cucumber juice, watercress, dill and soured cream, if using. Check seasoning and chill for four hours in the fridge.

5. Serve in bowls, garnished with parsley and a swirl of soured cream, if desired.

For Blood Stagnation

In clinic, this is an important time to work on Blood Stagnant types to get the Blood moving. Patients with endometriosis (see page 259) always come in mid-cycle and during their period.

I take two different approaches here: if you also have symptoms of Cold or Yang Deficiency we need some warming measures. So:

• Include warm foods in your diet, such as cardamom, cinnamon, fennel seed tea, thyme, basil, sage and rosemary.
• Use spices – try something different, perhaps Moroccan or Indian food?
• Make sure you eat *at least* one cooked meal a day.
• Use ginger – either in its powdered form or freshly peeled and sliced.(Alternatively, buy the preserved ginger in syrup: slice in half or thirds and pour boiling water on top; it is both warming and sweet and works well for sickness. Note: as ginger is Yang, Yin Deficient types and those with Heat need to avoid it.)

In pure Blood Stagnation types I suggest:

• abdominal massage using oils that will move Blood, such as cypress, lemon and geranium
• foods such as aubergine, leeks, saffron, turmeric and hawthorn berry
• paying special attention to physical and emotional movement now (and also outside of your fertile time) in order to keep a good healthy flow of blood.

Is the mind on board?

Affirmations

Say these morning and evening:

- 'My ovary easily releases an egg.'
- 'I am able to let go easily and freely and without any obstructions.'
- 'My ovaries are healthy and function perfectly.'
- 'My heart and mind are relaxed and I release an egg that is perfectly ripe.'
- 'My follicle has reached its perfect size. There is no obstruction to my releasing it now.'
- 'My Yin and Blood are at full growth and I will release a perfect egg with ease that will travel down my Fallopian tube to my uterus.'

Visualization

As I have already said, this is a fantastic time for visualization, particularly if you suffer from PCOS. My advice is to read the description of what is happening in your ovaries at the beginning of this chapter, then lie in a warm cosy place, where you are free from distractions, and really imagine it happening as you meditate. The affirmations will help too.

Try to visualize your ovary releasing the egg easily and freely; look at the illustration on page 201 and imagine it happening inside you. Imagine your body letting go, breathe freely and deeply and relax. PCOS patients need to be particularly mindful at this time and trust in their body's ability to produce and release an egg from the follicle at the correct time.

Qigong

infinity pattern

Stand with your feet hip-width apart, knees slightly bent. Your hands need to be held, palms down, at the level of your lower abdomen, below the navel. Sense the connection with the Qi of the earth; you can imagine you are absorbing it through the soles of your feet and through the palms of your hands.

Next, imagine the symbol of infinity: a figure eight, lying on its side. As you draw this symbol in your mind, feel the centre of it unite inside your lower abdomen. Feel the Qi move in all directions and on every level. Turn your hands over to face the sky (or one hand facing the sky and one facing the earth).

To close the practice, always return to the starting point with your palms facing the earth.

Yoga

The focus for yoga practice during ovulation is to release potential. In this phase of the cycle, the half-shoulder stand (see page 195) is enjoyable, and some of the more opening, liberating movements of the dog pose (see below) and its variations (number eight in the moon salute) are appropriate. Alternating the cobra (number seven in the moon salute) with dog can also be very strengthening and vitalizing at this time, and if you enjoy the camel pose (see page 193), include that in your programme too.

1. Dog Pose – Dog pose and the variations as described on page 342 are excellent at this point in the cycle. See the Appendix for a description of this pose.
2. Hare-Cobra – see page 342
3. Camel Pose (Ustrasana) – see Chapter Five for how to do this pose
4. If you experience pain on ovulation, these adaptations of the Hare Pose, described in the Appendix, may provide some relief: make two fists with your hands and settle them into the groin area before you fold forwards, to bring warmth and pressure into the ovaries; and/or place

a blanket over your lower back and have a friend hold
the ends of blanket firmly down either side of your hips,
bringing even pressure and warmth into the lower back.

If you are practising alone, then using the weight of a large
bag of pulses or beans on the lower back can have similar
benefits. If you don't have either of these then use a warm hot
water bottle on the lower back.

Meditation
For meditation practice, let the Heart/Womb *mudra* guide
your awareness within (see Chapter One).

Chapter Seven

Days 15–27: Implantation or PMT

For those trying to conceive, these two weeks can seem like the longest imaginable. I can tell you a thousand times not to stress in this phase, but even the most patient among you will have that creeping feeling of finger-drumming anticipation in your hearts right now. One of the reasons why I work in cycles is to spare my patients the agony of this wait and to take them out of that terrible lurch from ovulation to what one of them dubbed 'purgatory' and then their period.

I want you to practise mental strength, patience, meditation and yoga to help with this particular phase, when the preoccupation with conception can be all-consuming. Given the amount of activity that occurs between ovulation and the end of the cycle, it is worth investing every drop of your mental energy in remaining calm.

For those of you with obsessive tendencies, direct these into visualizations of the journey of the fertilized egg as outlined on page 201. This is the yang phase of the menstrual cycle. Yang is warming in essence, so it's imperative to support this warming process!

For others among you, this is the most dreaded part of

the cycle, *not* because you are thinking about conception, but because you suffer from Premenstrual Tension (PMT). I talk about PMT in detail in this chapter. It is worth knowing, however, that once they start concentrating on getting their cycle close to the 'ideal', most of my patients report that their premenstrual symptoms vanish almost completely. Nonetheless, you'll find tips here for coping with PMT and the yoga exercises and visualization will help with this too.

What's happening inside?

Days 15–22
The follicle that released the egg absorbs a fatty cholesterol called corpus luteum, which makes it turn an amber yellow colour. It continues to produce oestrogen and progesterone. These hormones prevent any of the other follicles from producing eggs.

Oestrogen and progesterone are crucial to very early pregnancy and will help maintain the egg if it is fertilized. In the uterus the endometrial lining is thickening and begins to produce nutrients in preparation for the blastocyst to implant.

Days 22–24
This is when you may experience the implantation of the egg. You may also experience a little blood spotting after implantation, which is sometimes confused with the onset of menstruation.

Days 25–27
If the egg is not fertilized, the corpus luteum disintegrates and is absorbed; oestrogen and progesterone drop, causing the built-up lining of the uterus to fall away as the menstrual flow.

Simultaneously, the pituitary gland starts to produce FSH and LH, which stimulate the ripening of the next cycle's eggs in the ovaries.

So, we covered ovulation in the last chapter and you may feel as if you were left with a bit of a cliffhanger: the egg has been released and can be fertilized any time within the next twenty-four hours. It will then complete its journey through the Fallopian tube and into the uterus where, around eight days after ovulation, it will implant. If the egg does not fertilize, it will be passed out, along with the endometrium (womb lining), in your menstrual bleed.

Implantation

As I said in an earlier chapter, the problems inherent in each 'type' can manifest at different points in the cycle. We have seen, for example, how Heat can shorten the follicular phase and how Damp can prevent ovulation.

At implantation, everyone has something to focus on: Blood Deficient types – because they need blood to build the womb lining; those with Yin Deficiency[1] (see page 138 on advanced states) – because of the quality of their eggs; Cold[2] types – because of the warmth needed to ensure implantation (hence the importance of a 'warm womb'); Damp types, because of excess mucus that can impede the progress of the fertilized egg; and those with Blood Stagnation because the 'sticky blood' doesn't clot well. Heat types also have the issue of 'reckless blood' (see page 138) to consider.

All these potential pitfalls explain why everything we have done up until now has been *so* important. We have been working to create the best soil for your beautiful plant. But what it also means is that you don't need to feel like a failure if this month is not the month that you conceive; you have another month to work on that soil so that it provides the very best environment for growth.

Premenstrual tension (PMT)

As we've established, hormones are responsible for the way you feel during your cycle. PMT is an umbrella term for a range of symptoms, the most common of which are cramps, backache, headache, the urge to cry, tiredness, depression and irritability. It is the most common reason for women to be off work in the UK, and it is estimated that up to 85 per cent of women experience at least one symptom of PMT.

These physical discomforts are caused in part by prosta-glandin hormones (which help regulate blood pressure, clotting and reproduction), produced in the uterus. They are essential for the menstrual cycle – but also for labour. They also travel through the bloodstream and can cause pain and discomfort elsewhere in the body.

Ovarian hormone levels also trigger symptoms through the brain's neurotransmitters, serotonin, noradrenaline and GABA (gamma-amino butyric acid), a central nervous system depressant. Changes in neurotransmitters, GABA and serotonin levels tend to be higher or lower than in those who don't experience bad PMT.

Around 10 per cent of women suffer from 'severe PMT' with additional symptoms; this is also termed premenstrual syndrome (PMS). Dr Katharina Dalton first described this in 1953, believing that these changes could be laid at the door of the hormone progesterone, which dips significantly before menstruation in all women in order to purge the uterine lining, and thus allow the cycle to start again. For those who have been trying to conceive for any length of time, it can be a double whammy: the arrival of the menstrual flow also represents the end of a time of anticipation and hope.

Dr Dalton devoted her life to monitoring the behaviour of women in the second half of their menstrual cycle. Her studies showed that the grades of schoolgirls dipped by 10 per cent before menstruation and that half of all female suicides in the 1950s and 1960s occurred in the four days before menstruation, as did half of all crimes committed by women. Women drivers, according to Dalton, were two and a half times more likely to have an accident before their period.[3]

In addition, Dr Dalton believed that in a small percentage of women, PMS was severe enough to cause a profound impact on their psychiatric health. She described this as 'a temporary psychosis' and even testified as an expert witness in the murder trials of women who had experienced severe PMS.[4]

Those who suffered worst were those in whom progesterone dipped the most and, therefore, those with the greatest hormone imbalance. She treated her patients and herself (she suffered with monthly migraines) with progesterone.

However, after tests revealed that the progesterone levels in those with PMS and those without were equal, she pursued another line of enquiry. She discovered that it was not just the universal dip in progesterone, but also its ability to *function* that exaggerated certain symptoms, and, she believed, this was related to food. Those who ate poorly saw their blood-sugar levels plunge, causing the body to release adrenalin. This interrupted the natural function of progesterone in the second half of the cycle. Her advice to patients was to apply the 'little and often' approach to meals, to prevent low blood sugar.

'This discovery has huge implications for fertility and miscarriage problems,' says Dr Marilyn Glenville, a nutritionist who specializes in fertility. She goes on to explain:
'If progesterone is blocked in this way it reduces the chances of maintaining a pregnancy, since [progesterone] is needed to

maintain the womb lining at the very start of pregnancy.

Many women who think they are infertile may therefore actually get pregnant without knowing it but lose the embryo early on because their bodies cannot use the progesterone they have. In such cases they may believe they are just having a normal period.'[5]

Today, we are left with a long legacy of negative attitudes towards menstruation, and even Dalton's heroic attempts to rescue us in some ways only serves to reinforce the entrenched view that women are all demented around the time of their period.

But it's crucial to remember that we *can* influence and regulate our cycles with alterations to our diet, exercise, general lifestyle and mental outlook. These practical changes will, in turn, effect a change in the way we experience our menstrual cycle.

As I have said before, one of the benefits of Chinese medicine is that it is almost always gentle and with few side effects. But Chinese medicine is not alone in suggesting natural remedies, such as diet, for period pains. One of the most effective supplements has been evening primrose oil, partly because it helps balance hormones and therefore treats the cause rather than the symptom. Evening primrose oil is an essential fatty

THE PILL AS TREATMENT FOR PAINFUL PERIODS

The contraceptive pill is often prescribed to young women with 'painful periods' as it removes period discomfort – but it does so by removing the reproductive cycle altogether, which is sort of like amputating your finger to release the pain of a cut. The Pill also comes with a risk of high blood pressure, thrombosis, cardiovascular disease and stroke. In my book, this makes it a fairly extreme option for the treatment of period pains.

CASE STUDY: LIVING WITH 'THE CURSE OF THE CURSE'

I had once had an amazing patient – a woman who really took everything I taught her about the menstrual cycle to heart. Her mother had never fully explained menstruation to her and had packed her off to boarding school where she was traumatized by the experience of her first period at which she felt shame and disgust. At boarding school, periods were known as 'the curse' and she always dreaded her premenstrual time.

She started to experience terrible premenstrual tension, which worsened over the years. In addition to the physical symptoms of PMT, she began to harbour intense feelings of resentment towards her husband and all those close enough to make demands on her time.

She described herself as 'a bit of a people pleaser', but said that the shadow of PMT would cause her to explode. I examined her: her tongue was very mauve and she sighed frequently as she described her situation. These symptoms are typical of Qi Stagnation. The sighing can be read as an attempt to 'free' the Qi that is clogged up in the chest. This can happen when people leave things unsaid and so they build up inside.

I felt that her symptoms were not so much related to progesterone or eating, but more to emotional issues. She had almost developed a fear of her periods that built up during the second half of her cycle. We did a lot of work on this fear and I suggested that she tried to adapt her life a little throughout the month. For example, if she did her socializing at the beginning of the cycle, she could reserve some time for herself as her cycle came full circle. I suggested that she use that time for more reflective pursuits, rather than start anything new.

During her worst days, I suggested gentle walks – perhaps by the river where she lived – but nothing too strenuous. Typically, patients with 'Stagnant' Qi try to do more premenstrually, which only adds to the problem in the long term. She came for regular acupuncture and she practised visualization, especially in the run-up to her period. Her favourite visualization was of a pretty, bubbling stream with a current. She would sit by this stream plucking the petals from a daisy and throwing them one by one into the water. The daisy petals represented her problems, and she would watch them bob away as the water carried them downstream. She told me that she could literally feel her problems leaving her body and travelling away with the water. She found this very empowering.

Gradually, her life was transformed. The PMT subsided as she learnt to become more positive about her 'time of the month'. Later, she substituted the visualizations with storytelling and has since become quite a talented writer.

acid (EFA). Foods that contain EFAs include sunflower seeds, olives, linseed, fish, rapeseed oil, walnut oil, sunflower oil and olive oil.

Other studies have shown the benefits of eating foods with a low glycaemic index (GI). This type of diet puts the emphasis on foods that will enter your bloodstream at a slow, even pace rather than causing a spike in blood sugar.

There are also gentle yoga stretches and breathing exercises (see pages 174–6) which can help with period pains.

Is the engine working?

For implantation to take place, three major things need to occur: a good quality embryo has to be produced, fertilization must take place and the womb lining has to be the correct thickness (8mm).

During the Yang phase, I treat those who are trying to conceive differently from those who are not. For those who are trying to conceive the treatment needs to be much gentler. I always assume conception has taken place, and my aim is to support the pregnancy, rather than try to rectify any tendencies. So, if someone has Cold tendencies I would still be warming them, but gently. If a patient has Heat, I would still keep her cool, but in a very toned-down way.

For those who are still working on rebalancing their systems, however, the treatment is stronger at this stage of the cycle. That's because this is the phase where we can really make a difference. If you are Blood Stagnant, I'll intensify the drive to move Blood because the run-up to your period provides an obvious exit for stagnated Blood, and also for Heat.

Q&A
Can I have my hair highlighted in early pregnancy?
The panel varied on this. However, on balance it was felt that due to the rapid growth and organ development in early pregnancy then it would be best avoided for the first 12 weeks.

Recommendations for everyone

Just as the first stage of the cycle needed moistening for everyone (except Damp), this stage needs warmth (except for Heat or Yin Deficient types). This is traditionally a time for 'warming the womb'. Western medicine often treats this phase of the cycle using progesterone, which also has a warming function. I recommend a 'kidney warmer'; you can make this yourself, using a cotton scarf tied comfortably round the waist with particular attention to the lower back. I also suggest you try:

- warming oils (except for Heat and those who may be pregnant)
- warming foods, such as ginger, little and often – don't let your blood sugar drop
- resting, as always in this process
- no vigorous exercise
- wearing socks in bed if it's cold outside
- avoiding sitting in draughts
- moxa on stomach 36 (see diagram, page 125 – Chapter Three), except for Heat and Yin Deficient types; this will help warm and build the Qi and Blood
- keeping your lower back warm – use a kidney warmer, as mentioned above.

CASE STUDY: GONE FISHING

Some months ago, I had a patient who was attempting to conceive. She was invited by friends on a fishing trip to Scotland where she realized, to her horror, she would be spending four days waist-high in cold water. Unable to get out of the commitment, she asked me what she should do.

I packed her off with a waterproof kidney warmer and some moxa sticks, which she carefully burned every night when she arrived back at base. She conceived that cycle.

- plenty of positive visualization, imagining exactly what is going on in the uterus.
- I suggest you try moxa; not directly above the abdomen, unless it is very cold to touch, but on the spleen channel of the lower leg – see diagram. By warming what is called 'the spleen channel', you can strengthen the 'holding and maintaining function' of what is termed the Spleen in Chinese medicine (which is not the same as the spleen in Western medicine). This is crucial at this stage of the cycle, and also for those who may be pregnant.

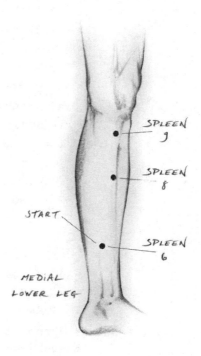

THE SPLEEN CHANNEL

SPLEEN 9

SPLEEN 8

START

SPLEEN 6

MEDIAL LOWER LEG

In the Yang phase I also concentrate on mental strength, with particular emphasis on banishing fear, so:

- Don't give in to fear and doubt or indulge bad thought – practise forgiveness.
- Practise daily affirmations.
- Step into your power: 'I am taking control of my life'.
- Transform fears into positives.
- Find your 'spark' – this is a good time for self-development.
- Find your inner strength and resilience.
- Use this as a time for quiet reflection.
- Consider and evaluate areas of your life that need change.

Finally, you should avoid:

- stress and overwork
- walking barefoot on cold floors
- getting too cold if you go swimming
- microwaves – steer well clear of these.

Is the fuel good?

Recommendations for everyone

- Limit your fruit intake (unless it is cooked with warming spices, e.g. apple baked with cinnamon).
- Slow-cook your food – baking and roasting vegetables is a good idea.
- Drink teas: chai, cinnamon, ginger or cardamom.
- Balance raw foods with something warm – so if you eat a salad, have a soup with it.
- Avoid cold drinks – drink water at room temperature.
- Avoid stodge (e.g. white carbohydrates).
- Avoid fats – except for monounsaturated and EFAs.

Store cupboard – for everyone except Heat

- Black beans
- Chestnuts
- Garlic
- Lamb
- Onions
- Pistachios
- Quinoa
- Raspberries
- Salmon
- Trout
- Walnuts

PINEAPPLES AND IMPLANTATION

Another easy food to include in your diet (for all but the most Damp types) is pineapple. Pineapples are high in the enzyme bromelain which may aid implantation due to its ability to thin the blood.

I suggest eating fresh pineapple (particularly the core if you can manage some of it); it is best eaten or juiced and then drunk on an empty stomach in order to aid absorption of the enzyme into the blood stream. Do not eat tinned pineapple since its levels of bromelain will have been destroyed through the heating and tinning process. Don't overdo it: one serving or one glass of freshly squeezed juice a day post-ovulation is ample.

For Cold

Touch your tummy below the navel. Is it cold? If you are experiencing a high level of Cold at this stage of the cycle it may affect your chances to incubate the embryo – and as I tell my patients, 'You can't grow a baby in a fridge'. Take a hot-water bottle (not too hot), wrap it in a towel and hold it to your lower abdomen as you lie and relax on your bed. If possible, do this for forty minutes towards the end of the day, between 4 and 6 p.m. – unless you think you may be pregnant, in which case you can use the moxa on the Spleen Channel, as described on page 225.

As I've said, warmth is crucial in this phase and the notion of 'a warm womb for conception' is a basic principle in the treatment of fertility in China. In addition to all the recommendations above:

- Use Moxa on stomach 36, or see a practitioner for acupuncture.
- Use warming oils in the bath.

For Damp

Damp makes it hard for the egg to implant because it clogs its passage through the Fallopian tubes with damp and phlegm, slowing its progress and therefore 'missing' its window for implantation.

Like Cold types, Damp types need to warm their bodies to expel the excess water, which may cause bloating or diarrhoea. Chinese dietary therapy recommends several ingredients to help dispel Cold from the stomach, which Damp types can also use. These include dried ginger, cinnamon and dried orange peel. Cinnamon and ginger can be ground into a powder and used in cooking or taken in a tea, and will relieve abdominal swelling. Dried ginger is more effective than fresh for this purpose. Orange peel can be used in stews and soups or powdered for use in cooking or teas. It will also relieve other congestion or indigestion.

Soya beans and bean curd are also recommended for all Damp people, whether their problem is due to Damp/Heat or Damp/Cold, because these beans strengthen the 'Spleen' and help it to deal with the issue of Damp.

Too much Damp can impede the passage of the egg through the Fallopian tubes, so that it arrives too late for implantation and the endometrium has already started to shed.

Many patients find it helpful to visualize the egg travelling down the Fallopian tubes with ease, arriving at an endometrium that is receptive and well nourished.

For Damp/Heat

Chinese medicine recommends the following for the treatment of Damp/Heat:

- green tea
- mung beans
- bean sprouts (cooked not raw)
- millet porridge.

For Blood Deficient

This stage is, of course, crucial to Blood Deficient types because an endometrium that is less than 8mm thick will not support implantation. See the advice recommended for everyone above, but take special care with the following:

- Don't overwork.
- Don't get stressed.
- REST!
- Nourish yourself with foods that suit any other tendency you may have.
- Practise exercise for mental stillness – Blood Deficient types are often strung out and tired and prone to emotional upheaval, which is particularly dangerous in this phase.

- Visualize your endometrium at the perfect thickness, with a rich supply of blood to receive your fertilized embryo.

Note: it takes at least four cycles to get on track, so even if you are not trying to conceive visualize this anyway.

For Heat

Heat is the anomaly in this phase of the cycle. We need to cool Heat and prevent what I call 'reckless blood' (see page 138). Try to do the following:

- meditate
- concentrate on calming the mind and cooling the blood
- acupressure on the points around the knee and above the knee
- eat carefully – see suggestions below
- visualize something cool – such as a walk on a snowy mountainside – this may help to regulate the system.

In addition, if you are generating a lot of heat – you are agitated and sweaty, for example – try placing a cooling gel pack from fridge behind the knee. The traditional Chinese medicine view was that pregnancies failed because of the Womb not being warm enough at implantation. Increasingly in modern practice, however, I am seeing Heat patients who get excessively heated in the city, perhaps due to the overheating of our environment today. Also, we don't understand how to moderate our mental and physical activities, and this generates a lot of internal Heat. That's why you really do need to keep your cool. Supercharged Heat impedes the flow of blood, particularly around implantation.

Q&A

Can I go in the sun in early pregnancy?
Many pregnant women find that their body will tell them what is good for them. You may well be more sensitive and less tolerant of the sun than normal. Avoid long exposure to the sun and slathering yourself in oil and baking yourself, it will heat your blood!

For Qi and Blood Stagnation

Qi Stagnant patients may experience contractions in the abdomen and Fallopian tubes, inhibiting the smooth flow of the egg into the uterus.

Those prone to Blood Stagnation may have sticky Blood, which is problematic if the embryo is to implant successfully. Blood Stagnation may manifest in the form of fibroids, polyps, endometriosis, or just a general poor circulation of blood in the abdomen. Concentrate on a smooth flow of blood in visualizations along with affirmations.

If you suspect that you may have an advanced case of Blood Stagnation, look under your tongue and see how distended the veins are. You may need to suspend trying for a baby until you have corrected it. Acupuncture and herbal medicine are excellent for a moderate case of Blood Stagnation and to remove any significant blocks to implantation (see Resources, page 357, for practitioners). More advanced cases that do not respond to this first-line treatment, however, may call for intervention (see Chapter Eight). Don't give up on following the plan though, as it all helps.

Avoiding alcohol and sugar premenstrually is important for those with Qi Stagnation as it is a lethal mix in terms of mood.

Premenstrual – Blood and Qi-moving foods

The following are all useful for getting Blood and Qi moving.
- Fish: crayfish,* prawns,* shrimp,* crab*
- Fruit: plums, peaches
- Vegetables: radishes, leeks, celery, brown seaweed, aubergines, spring onions, onions
- Nuts and seeds
- Spices and herbs: ginger, garlic, pepper, marjoram, coriander, chilli, turmeric, mustard leaf
- Other: vinegar, brown sugar

Note: Foods marked with an asterisk are best avoided by those who may have conceived.

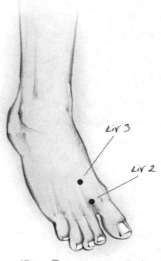

ACUPRESSURE POINTS ON THE FOOT

Liv 3

Liv 2

TOP AND LATERAL FOOT

Acupressure for Qi Stagnation

The key acupressure point to release Qi Stagnation is on the top of the foot between your big and second toes (see diagram, right). When you apply pressure, you may notice that it is fairly sensitive. Actually, the level of discomfort often reflects the levels of stagnation. It is a wonderful point to use premenstrually. I often joke to patients that they will be much nicer after I have needled the point and that they won't remember what they were feeling cross about. It's true – it really does dissolve tension and irritability.

Yoga for Qi Stagnation

Yoga will also help with the physical symptoms of Qi Stagnation; it is perfect, as it works all the areas where tension collects and it frees the flow of Qi in the meridian.

Try to bring some awareness into your life – ask yourself: what are your triggers? and what winds you up at this time? And give yourself a break – don't do things you don't want to and then moan about it; have the courage to say 'No' in the first place. You'll be doing everyone a favour in the long run!

For more on yoga and asking yourself questions, see the 'Is the mind on board?' section below.

Is the mind on board?

In the luteal phase you are often more in tune with your needs, so this is a good time for inward-looking activities. It is thought that emotional issues that arise during this time

Spicy Prawn & Aubergine Curry

A great recipe for Qi and Blood Stagnation. Not recommended if you may have conceived.

Serves 4

For the red Thai curry paste
8 dry red chillies, deseeded
1 tsp ground coriander seeds
½ tsp ground cumin
1 tsp ground white pepper
4 cloves garlic, chopped
2 lemongrass stalks, chopped
1 handful chopped coriander
1 tsp kaffir lime leaves
2.5cm piece galangal, chopped
2 tsp shrimp paste
2 tsp vegetable oil
1 tsp salt
For the prawn and aubergine curry
1 tbsp oil
1 garlic clove
1 tbsp red Thai curry paste
300ml tin coconut milk (or 200ml crème fraîche)
2 tbsp fish sauce
1 tbsp fine brown sugar
1 tsp turmeric
2 fresh lemongrass stalks, bruised with the blunt edge of a knife
300ml fish stock (organic cubes will do) or water
1 medium-sized aubergine, cut into chunks

salt
400g peeled raw prawns (or 200g prawns and 200g salmon, cut into bite-sized chunks)
3 handfuls fresh spinach
juice of ½ lime
fresh coriander, to garnish

1. To make the Thai curry paste, grind all the ingredients in a mortar and pestle or put in a blender and blitz until combined into a paste. (If all this sounds too much like hard work, a pot of organic red Thai curry paste will do the trick!)

2. To make the curry, heat the oil in a pan and sauté the chopped garlic until brown. Add the curry paste and cook over a low heat for a couple of minutes.

3. Whisk in the coconut milk or crème fraîche, then gradually add the fish sauce, sugar, turmeric, lemongrass and fish stock and simmer for about 5 minutes.

4. While the sauce is simmering, chop the aubergine into chunks and sprinkle with salt, rinse thoroughly and add to the curry sauce. Simmer for 5 to 10 minutes or until the aubergine chunks are tender.

5. Set the curry aside. When ready to serve, reheat the sauce and when it starts to boil, add the peeled and washed prawns (and salmon, if using) and spinach and stir until all the spinach leaves have wilted and the prawns are cooked (approximately 2–3 minutes). Squeeze in the lime.

6. Serve garnished with chopped coriander.

are the areas of your life that need tending to, so do not ignore them. It is important that you make space for some inward connection and reflective work with some of the ideas throughout this book. You will not be feeling quite so expansive as in the follicular phase, which is the 'creation phase' of the cycle. As you near the time of your period it is an idea to go out less and spend time organizing things at home. This will help you feel grounded and settled.

Affirmations

Say these in the morning and evening:
- 'I am not held back by fear or doubt.'
- 'My courage is strong, my heart is strong, I feel together and calm.'
- 'I have stepped into my power. I have taken charge of my fertility.'

Visualization

Christiane Northrup says that, 'under hypnosis a woman who is given positive suggestions about her menstrual cycle will be less apt to suffer from menstruation-related symptoms'.[6]

She quotes a study in which women who were not premenstrual were told they were and automatically felt the adverse side effects associated with the menstrual phase, such as cramps, irritability and water retention. Another group was told that they were not premenstrual when they were and their symptoms lifted.

This goes some way to show just how much we are influenced by suggestion. We do have the power to alter the way we feel with thought. Try visualizing any premenstrual symptoms falling away and leaving you feeling clear and 'light'.

Qigong

This is a qigong exercise for the post-ovulation, implantation phase, called 'Nourish and Implant the foetus'.

There are two positions in which you can do this exercise. Either sit with your legs crossed and your heel pressing into your perineum, or kneeling with your legs crossed beneath you and your heel pressing into your perineum.

1. Make a fist with your right hand and then put your left thumb into the centre of your fist, making sure you can touch the centre of your palm. This is the acupuncture point Heart Protector 8.

2. Hold both hands against your lower abdomen, and imagine you are holding the power of your lower belly in your hands. Now imagine you are sending power and energy into the uterus and the pelvis.

3. Try this pose for 20 minutes in the morning and evening. If you can, try to meditate in this pose, or use it to visualise implantation.

Yoga

Let the focus of your yoga practice during the premenstrual phase be to nourish and grow. The gentle but rhythmic repetition of the *shakti bandha* (stirring the porridge, see page 338, Appendix) can help to dissipate any physical congestion. Be sure to allow a sufficient rest period and, if you are feeling edgy, use this powerful adaptation of the full yogic breath to release physical and mental tension:

1. Golden thread breathing

The golden thread works well in any position, but be aware that if you practise lying down you are likely to fall asleep. Tune into a gentle pattern of breathing that is effortless. Take an extra yawn, release your jaw, throat and teeth.

Allow there to be a very small space between your top and bottom teeth, top and bottom lip: just enough that you might imagine a piece of tissue paper held between the lips, such a

CASE STUDY: ME

I am the case study this time. There have been a couple of occasions in my life when I have needed to find my way through difficult issues. At such times, I've learnt that taking a good look at yourself in the bathroom mirror can help you be honest with yourself and gain some spiritual strength.

Once you face the truths within you, you can start working towards jettisoning the parts of your life that are harming you and building up your inner self-belief. You may even find that gradually, you can begin to do your affirmations while looking yourself dead in the eye in the bathroom mirror – although, you might find it a little disconcerting at first. (My husband caught me doing this once; at the time he thought I had lost my marbles, but I think he's used to it now!)

small gap that it is practically invisible. Breathe in through your nose. Breathe out between slightly parted lips. Feel a fine, cool breeze passing out between your lips. Concentrate on relaxing your cheeks, lips and face. Don't purse your lips; feel them soft. Feel your breath travelling in through your nose, and out through your mouth. Allow the breath to be so fine that it feels as if a fine golden thread is spinning out between your lips. It's a thin, golden thread, like embroidery yarn, smooth and silky, spinning out with every exhalation.

Allow each exhalation to lengthen, without forcing, but simply letting the out breath increase in length, as the golden thread of breath spins out into the air in front of you. With each inhalation, allow for your breath to go in through your nose and feel the breeze of exhalation travelling between your lips, into the air in front of your closed eyes. Let the end of the golden thread carry your mental attention further and further away with each exhalation.

The heart of this practice is softness. You are not pursing the lips or making them tight as if to whistle. The lips are soft and the breath passing between them is silent and gentle. The lengthening of the exhalation is achieved effortlessly: simply because the gap through which the breath passes is so tiny, it takes a long time for all the breath to get out. There is no sense of force; simply watch the breath lengthen, following it out into the space in front of you. It should feel completely comfortable and soothing. If you are struggling to exhale because the gap is too small, simply widen the gap.

Any exhalation is an antidote to pain and tension. The golden thread's extended exhalation makes this antidote more powerful. The longer the exhalation, the greater the distance is between mind and body. Allow the golden thread of the breath to travel out as far as is comfortable for you, and let the body make a voyage back to its natural healing state of easeful rest. When the mental awareness is at the far end of the long exhalation, then the body can rest.

2. Breath-balancing pose (padadhirasana)

Balancing breaths can help to cope with the demands of mood swings or turbulent emotions. Use them at the end of your yoga programme, just before the meditation.

This is a simple way to develop breath awareness and a balanced flow of breath in the nostrils; it promotes an even, measured pattern of breath and helps to create a calm and attentive frame of mind.

Sit on your heels or on a bolster or cushion to support the kneeling posture comfortably. With a straight spine, let your shoulders drop away from your ears. With your hands resting on your thighs, watch the breath for seven rounds as you establish a full yogic inhalation and exhalation (see page 336). When the breath is rhythmic and even, cross your arms over your chest, tucking your right thumb under your left armpit and your left thumb under your right armpit. Work your thumbs up high into the warmth of your armpits, then let your elbows drop down towards your waist.

Close your eyes and focus your attention on the flow of

breath into and out of the nostrils. Be aware of a triangular pattern of breath, as the air flows into the nostrils and up the sides of your nose to the tip of the triangle at the point between your eyebrows. Be aware of that same triangle as the breath flows down from the bridge of your nose to your nostrils. When you are ready, release your thumbs from under your armpits and rest the backs of your hands on your thighs. Observe the pattern of the flow of breath in the nostrils. Note any changes that may have occurred.

3. Alternate-nostril breath (nadi shodana pranayama)

This is a calming and quietening breath to balance the flow in the nostrils. It promotes tranquillity and ease. Begin by sitting comfortably, observing your breath, then establish a full yogic breath. Aim to allow the rhythm of this complete breath to continue throughout the practice of alternate-nostril breathing. Raise your right hand to your face, with right shoulder relaxed and right elbow dropped. Rest your index and middle fingers of your right hand on the point between your eyebrows. Rest your right thumb lightly on your right nostril and your right ring finger lightly on the left nostril. Let the little finger be free, and check that you can use the index and middle fingers as a pivot, alternately opening and closing the right and left nostrils with the thumb and ring finger.

Establish a relaxed rhythm of full yogic breathing. Close the left nostril with your ring finger and allow your breath to come in through the right nostril. At the end of the inhalation, switch nostrils by closing your right nostril with your right thumb and allow the breath to leave through the left nostril. At the end of the exhalation, keep your right nostril closed with your thumb and draw the next inhalation through the left nostril. At the end of that inhalation, switch nostrils by closing your left nostril with the ring finger and allow the breath to leave through the right nostril. That is one complete round.

For additional practice, see the core sequence in Chapter One the Appendix.

Note: remember not to invert if you think you may be pregnant or if your period has started.

For those who find out they are pregnant

You are pregnant! Congratulations! This is the fabulous event you have been waiting for. I think it is important to allow yourself to feel thrilled – even if you are also a little nervous. For many women, this is a major breakthrough and the end of a very long journey in fertility.

In our mothers' day, many women waited until they had missed three periods before believing that they were indeed pregnant. With the methods of testing we have today, however, most women know pretty much immediately if they have conceived with the aid of a simple test from the chemist. This can bring mixed blessings. The wait to tell friends and family may feel agonizingly long, as is the journey through the rocky period of early pregnancy when there are still high risks involved.

It is a nerve-wracking time, but it's also a beautiful one. You've had a lot of practice with patience; you need to just eke out all the brilliant work you've done so far for a few more weeks.

My advice is: take it easy and look after yourself. Hold on to your inward smile and try to stay calm. Book an appointment with the doctor as soon as you can, especially if you have had previous complications and if you are likely to need a six- or eight-week scan. Continue to take folic acid supplements and please be aware of those foods you need to avoid during pregnancy, such as raw eggs, raw meat, pâtés and soft cheeses. (For more information visit *http://www.eatingfor-pregnancy.org.uk* and *www.nhs.uk/pregnancy*.) In terms of my baby-making plan and your 'type', you should continue to *avoid* foods that exacerbate your type, but it's as important to *include* the foods that help reduce the effects of a type.

Remember, everything you do needs to be gentle, gentle, gentle. Avoid all essential oils at this stage of your pregnancy and exercise needs to be light: try walks and gentle yoga and breathing. Don't take any medication unless you have cleared it with your GP or obstetrician first.

Use the meditation you have been practising up until now. And remember the connection between the Heart and the Womb and how important it is to keep working on it (see the exercise with one hand on the heart and the other on the womb, page 350).

Fear

Those of you who have had an especially complicated journey up to this point may find it hard to be positive, even after seeing the positive pregnancy test. For this reason, I feel it is vital to keep 'hope in the heart' and not to let fear creep in.

My view is that you are where you are now, at this moment, and nobody can take this moment away from you. None of us knows what is around the corner; we can only ever truly be in the moment. You need to keep the strong image of yourself holding your baby or, if you prefer, your pregnant bump. Hold it really firmly in your mind and allow yourself to feel hope.

Affirmations for pregnancy

- 'I am pregnant now and I allow this pregnancy to take place easily.'
- 'I am happy and secure with this pregnancy.'
- 'I allow myself to feel confident with my newly pregnant body.'
- 'With each new day I am growing in confidence.'
- 'Every day in every way it's getting better and better.'

For those who are not yet pregnant

Stay positive! Continue to follow the cycles and read the next chapter. And remember, it takes the average couple nine months to conceive. Instead of viewing it as a failure this month, see this as an opportunity to spend more time preparing the 'soil' and cultivating great health. There is still plenty you can do to prepare for a healthy conception on my baby-making programme. Make sure you are fully committed to the plan, with your heart and your head fully on board.

Part III

THE BABY-MAKING PLAN FOR ASSISTED CONCEPTION

Chapter Eight

'Why am I not getting pregnant?'

At this point, the big questions for those of you who have been trying to conceive for a while will be: why are you not getting pregnant and when should you ask for help? And there are no general answers to these.

For a start, everyone's fertility journey will have been different up to this point. You may have been trying for two years or for six months. You may even have been trying for less time than that, but are concerned about your age or an existing gynaecological issue.

Taking the decision to go to the doctor can feel like a daunting one, but it doesn't have to be. In this process, you'll constantly need to reassess your goals (actually, this is great skill to learn for parenting!). It could be that the doctor's reassurance gives you renewed confidence to keep trying; or preliminary tests may give you a clean bill of health and, in turn, give you renewed confidence to keep trying. A gynaecologist colleague told me that it always amazes him how many couples fall pregnant the cycle after seeing him for the first time, with no treatment whatsoever. Sometimes the cry for help is, in itself, a solution.

All that being said, age is a factor in considering when to ask for help. If you are in your mid-twenties and have been trying for a few months, there may not be any urgency, and I would advise such a couple to have a fertility plan in place if they had not conceived after nine months. This might be, for example, to try for a year using natural methods and complementary medicine, supported with Western medicine diagnostics after one year, such as a monitored cycle (a diagnostic cycle in which scans and blood tests are performed throughout to identify potential problems).

'INFERTILITY PATIENTS' – DISCARDING THE LABEL

One thing I often hear in clinic is how patients have gone from the 'nothing's happening' stage, to being classed as 'infertility patients', merely because they picked up the phone and asked for a referral. Clearly this is not a label that anyone wants. It can feel scary and even pushes some couples back into the shadows of not seeking help. My advice is to treat the label as just that, and not as an 'identity'.

If, however, you are already thirty-five, waiting two years before you start a family may be too long. If you and your partner came to me and said you'd been trying for six months, had already done my pre-conception plan for four cycles and were both seemingly in good health, I would say it's time to get tested.

At age thirty-eight, fertility takes the biggest plunge. From then on, the issue of time becomes a significant factor. At this point, I would say that testing becomes a priority, especially if both partners are healthy and not smoking or drinking alcohol.

I should add here that if you have already had a gynaecological issue diagnosed, such as polycystic ovaries or endometriosis, it may take longer for you to conceive and may be a factor in deciding how long you are willing to try to conceive naturally before seeking help with fertility medicine.

And, of course, it is not just women who can have an issue with fertility. Male subfertility can be an issue in around 30 per cent or more cases of infertility.

What is Infertility?

Infertility, as defined by the National Institute for Health and Clinical Excellence (NICE), is the failure 'to get pregnant after two years of regular unprotected sex'. It is, according to government figures, the most common reason for women in the UK aged twenty to forty-five to see their GP. It affects between one in six and one in seven couples in Britain – approximately 3.5 million people – at some point in their fertility journey. Although the majority of these women will become pregnant naturally (without fertility medicine) given time, a significant minority will not.

Fertility testing

The emotional side of testing

Testing is a double-edged sword. On the one hand, many couples need clarity at some point in their fertility journey. On the other, the process is extremely stressful.

You may already be feeling under par because of months of trying for a pregnancy. It can be frustrating and confusing. You may find that it dents your self-confidence in all areas, or that it exacerbates underlying feelings of low self-esteem. You may also harbour feelings of resentment towards friends who have had no problem conceiving.

Stress, as well as being a by-product of this situation, can also make it worse. So, in this chapter I'm going to help you navigate the rollercoaster journey of tests and test results and make it as stress-free as possible.

I'd like you to continue to refer to all the tools we have discussed thus far

Q&A

I have been told that I have an abnormal shaped uterus. Can I still conceive naturally? Natural conception is possible in 65–75 per cent of women with this problem.

– meditation, visualization, affirmations, yoga and positive-thinking techniques – to keep you steady. And don't give up!

At the GP

No two couples are the same and no two fertility journeys are the same. There is a whole range of factors that can be implicated, which is why, perhaps, so many people ask for help outside of the normal system which does not address all of these. And why people come to practitioners like me, often before they see their GP or private specialist.

However, my approach is not to act as GP. I have taken you through the process that I use in my clinic, and now we are going to look at the issues that arise in the Western medical system. Don't feel daunted – think of it as being empowering, as it will arm you with the information you'll need as you take the first steps down this route.

It is important that you find a GP (or specialist if you are going the private route) who really listens to you. And if you are not happy with the information you are given, seek a second opinion. Don't be afraid of the system. Time is precious when it comes to fertility and if you *feel* something is wrong, you owe it to yourself to follow your instincts.

FERTILITY FACTS AND FIGURES

Of 100 couples of all ages trying to conceive naturally:

- 20 per cent will conceive within one month of the remainder, 70 per cent will conceive within six months of the remainder, 85 per cent will conceive within a year of the remainder, 90 per cent will conceive within eighteen months.
- Ninety-five per cent of the original 100 couples will have conceived within two years.

The age factor

As we know, women become less fertile with age (the effect of age on male fertility is less clear):

- Around 95 per cent of women over thirty-five who have regular, unprotected sex will get pregnant after three years of trying.
- Only 75 per cent of women aged thirty-eight will do so.

Causes of infertility

The following reasons for infertility were collected from patient registration forms for IVF treatment[1]:

- Male factor – 32.5 per cent
- Female factor – 32.5 per cent
- Multiple male and female factors – 10.8 per cent
- Unexplained – 23.1 per cent
- Other factors – 1.1 per cent

Questions the GP might ask you
General
- How old are you?
- How much do you weigh (see Body Mass Index, page 56)?
- How long have you been trying?
- Are your periods regular? Are they heavy?
- Do you bleed in between your cycles or after intercourse?
- Do you experience pain in your menstrual cycle?
- How often do you have sex? Is it painful?
- Do you take any medication?
- Are you aware of any other medical issues, such as thyroid problems, anaemia or diabetes?
- Is there any relevant family medical history?

Sexual history
- How many partners have you had?
- What contraceptives have you used – e.g. the Pill, the coil, condoms etc?
- Have you had any sexually transmitted diseases (STDs, see box, page 250)?

Pregnancy history
- Have you had previous pregnancies (and how did they end, i.e. live birth, ectopic, termination, miscarriage, etc.)?
- How many miscarriages have you experienced?
- Have you had any operations, such as a Caesarean section or an appendicectomy?
- Have you experienced any pregnancy-related complications?

Lifestyle
- What is your profession?
- What are your working hours?
- What are your stress levels like?

- How often do you exercise?
- Do you smoke?
- How much alcohol do you drink?
- Do you take recreational drugs?
- What is your diet like?

Questions you might want to ask the GP
I recommend that you work out what you both want from your meeting with the GP. It may be that one of you just wants to find out that all is in working order, while the other wants to press ahead with finding out about fertility medicine as soon as possible. My colleague, consultant obstetrician Michael Dooley, says that patients' criteria for seeing him tend to fall under the following four main headings:

- They want to find out why they are not getting pregnant.
- They want to find out why they are not getting pregnant and they would also like a pregnancy.
- They would like a pregnancy and would also like to find out why they are not getting pregnant.
- They don't mind why they are not getting pregnant; they just want a pregnancy.[2]

I think it's an idea to work out which description fits you best. This will give you a goal to work towards with the GP.

Q&A
I have lots of discharge which sometimes makes my vagina itchy and sore, then it clears up but it keeps coming back. Is this normal?
It sounds like you have have a vaginal infection which will need to be treated by your G.P. It is important that your partner is tested as well as it is easy to keep passing infections back and forth between you. Some infections give very mild symptoms which seem to clear up and then come back so it can be confusing. As a rule if there is itching, discoloration or a strange smell it is always worth getting your G.P. to take a swab.

SEXUALLY TRANSMITTED DISEASES THAT IMPACT ON FERTILITY

A sexually transmitted disease (or STD, also known as sexually transmitted infection or STI) is an infection that is spread through sexual contact. If there is any remote chance you may have one, you must get it checked out, just to be on the safe side.

STDs affect fertility primarily through the upper genital tract in women, but some also affect male fertility. In the UK, sexually transmitted diseases are a growing problem and the latest NHS statistics show that the two most common ones, chlamydia and gonorrhoea have leapt by 150 per cent and 42 per cent respectively in the last ten years.

The best way to prevent an STD is by practising safe sex. Some STDs have no outward symptoms, so the only sure way to check if you have one is to get tested. Chlamydia, for example, can wreak havoc in your reproductive system without you knowing – until you try to conceive.

Below, I discuss only those STDs that can impact on your fertility. So, I do not tackle genital herpes, HIV, AIDS or syphilis. For more information on these diseases see *www.nhs.gov.uk.*

CHLAMYDIA

A screening programme in 2006 revealed that at least one in ten under 25s in the UK is infected with chlamydia, a bacterial infection, which is the most common and fastest-spreading STD. But the true figure may be much higher. It is often called the 'silent STD' because it can have no early symptoms. The UK government is encouraging young men and women who may be at risk from the disease to get checked early. Left untreated, chlamydia can cause infertility in both men and women.

Symptoms
In women symptoms can include:
- cystitis – a stinging sensation on urinating
- unusual vaginal discharge
- pain in the lower abdomen – caused by pelvic inflammatory disease (PID) – this is sometimes mistaken for something else
- pain on intercourse
- bleeding or spotting between periods, or bleeding after intercourse
- Bartholin's abscess.

Or there may be no symptoms at all.

In men symptoms can include:

- a stinging sensation on urinating
- unusual clear discharge from the penis (this is the most common sign)
- an inflamed urethra
- pain or tenderness around the testicles
- discomfort at the tip of the penis that subsides after a few days; once the pain has subsided, many men assume the infection has gone and they don't seek medical attention – unfortunately, however, the infection is still present
- painful joints.

Diagnosis

A swab of the cells in the area of infection (cervix or penis) is taken and then tested.

Treatment

In its early stages, chlamydia can be treated with antibiotics. A further swab may be taken to ensure the treatment has worked. In advanced cases, women may need IVF in order to conceive (see page 287).

Complications

In women:

- Pelvic inflammatory disease (PID), also know as pelvic infection.
- Damage to the Fallopian tubes, preventing the egg from travelling to the uterus.
- Increased risk of ectopic pregnancy because the fertilised egg cannot travel to the uterus and thus implants in the Fallopian tube. The tube can then rupture causing bleeding – which can be life-threatening.
- If natural conception does occur, there is a risk of passing the infection on to the newborn infant during childbirth.

In men:

- Inflammation of the testicles and of the tubes that deliver sperm, causing pain, swelling and redness on the scrotum.
- In rare cases, the infection can trigger joint inflammation, which is difficult to treat.

GONORRHOEA

Gonorrhoea is a fast-growing bacteria that multiplies in moist, warm areas such as the cervix, urethra, mouth or rectum. Like chlamydia, the disease can spread to the uterus and Fallopian tubes, causing PID and leading to infertility. In 50 per cent of women and 33 per cent of men there are no visible symptoms at all. If symptoms do develop, it is usually within a week of contact, although patients may be infected for months without visible signs.

Symptoms
In women symptoms can include:
- burning pain on urinating
- unusual discharge: sometimes yellowish or bloody in colour
- bleeding or spotting between periods
- mild lower-abdominal pain (PID).

Or there may be no symptoms at all.

In men symptoms can include:
- burning sensation on urinating
- yellow discharge from the penis.

Diagnosis
A swab taken by your doctor can determine whether you have the disease.

Treatment
Antibiotics, then another swab is needed to ensure the infection has gone.

Complications
In women:
- The infection can lead to PID.
- The Fallopian tubes can become blocked, leading to infertility or ectopic pregnancy.
- The infection can be passed on to the newborn baby during delivery (and it can result in blindness).

In men:
- Inflammation of the epididymis – the tube at the top and sides of the testicles where sperm passes.

GENITAL WARTS

Genital warts are very contagious.

Symptoms
In women symptoms can include:
- fleshy, raised growths with cauliflower-like appearance on the inside or outside of the vagina, the cervix and the anus
- itching in this area.

Symptoms are not always visible, however, and even when they are, they may also disappear.

In men symptoms can include:
- fleshy, raised growths on the tip and/ or shaft of the penis, the scrotum or around the anus; the warts may appear in tiny clusters but can grow into large masses.

In some cases there are no visible symptoms. And symptoms may also disappear, while the virus remains.

Diagnosis
Genital warts are diagnosed by a physical examination.

Treatment
The warts can be removed by freezing, burning or by laser treatment. They can be treated with topical creams or lotions.

Complications
Genital warts do not cause fertility problems, but women with warts are more likely to have an STD such as chlamydia.

What are the basic fertility tests?

In most cases your GP will do the tests, but you may be referred to a gynaecologist. First, your GP will perform a physical examination, in which they may check your weight and look for:

- abnormal hair growth (which may indicate PCOS)
- skin conditions (such as acne, which may also indicate PCOS)
- changes in voice, indicating hormonal changes
- an enlarged thyroid
- any abdominal scarring, which may impede implantation.

The GP may offer you a pelvic examination to check the structure of the reproductive system; they will also check your vagina, cervix, uterus and ovaries. They will be looking for tenderness, inflammation, nodules or masses, irregular bleeding, vaginal discharge or immobility in the uterus. Your doctor should ask you about any abnormalities in the vagina cervix or uterus, such as tightness or pain. This will provide evidence of:

- fibroids
- endometriosis
- infection
- abnormal structure.

A blood test – for your follicle-stimulating hormone (FSH) levels – is taken on Day 2 to 4 of your cycle and it's an indicator of how hard the brain has to work to produce the egg, or as my gynaecologist colleague Jeannie Yoon explains, 'This is how hard the engine has to work to keep the car running.' A higher FSH may be indicative of a poor ovarian reserve and/or ovarian function. To be referred to the NHS for IVF, most clinics will want your FSH level to be under ten (ten and over being considered elevated). However, many private hospitals will still undertake treatment if it's ten or over. For help with lowering your FSH levels, see page 294.

Note: FSH doesn't tell the full story, so having a low FSH level doesn't automatically mean that you'll face an obstacle-free path to pregnancy. So, just concentrating on the FSH result is the equivalent of only looking through one window of a house and deciding you have enough information to buy it.

There is a second test, called an AMH test, which checks for levels of anti-Mullerian hormone. This is more an indicator of quantity or 'how much fuel is left in the tank'.

When will you be referred to a specialist?

Again, there is no simple answer. Generally speaking, if you have an underlying condition, you are over thirty-eight or your test results reveal an abnormality, you may be referred promptly. You can also ask for a referral. Otherwise, your GP may ask you to come back if nothing has happened after a few months.

Invasive tests – tubal problems

One of the first invasive tests that your doctor may suggest is one to assess any damage to your Fallopian tubes. This is a common cause of infertility and affects between 20 and 25 per cent of those seeking fertility treatment. It can be due to a whole range of factors and impacts on your ability to conceive in a number of ways.

Damage to the tiny hairs (cilia) that help the egg's passage to the uterus can reduce their function and thus the ability of the egg to move down the Fallopian tube. Damage to the cilia can prevent the sperm from reaching the egg, therefore reducing the chance of fertilization. And a block in the tube can stop the egg from being fertilized or the fertilized egg from reaching the uterus (this increases the risk of ectopic pregnancy, which is where the fertilized egg embeds in the Fallopian tube rather than the uterus).

These problems may be caused by:
- an infection in the pelvic area
- previous ectopic pregnancy
- any surgery in the area, such as an appendicectomy, termination of pregnancy, birth or miscarriage
- an ovarian cyst
- abdominal surgery which can occasionally cause scarring
- the spread of an infection from other organs, such as a ruptured appendix
- infection from a coil that spreads to the tubes
- STDs, such as chlamydia and gonorrhoea (see page 250).

Symptoms include:
- bad period pains
- irregular periods
- heavy bleeding
- bleeding between periods
- bleeding after intercourse
- tenderness in the pelvic area.

There may also be no symptoms at all.

The simplest and most common way to check for tubal damage is to have an HSG (hysterosalpingogram). This is when dye is injected through the cervix and an X-ray picture is taken of the womb and Fallopian tubes to identify any problems. Tubal damage may also be investigated using a procedure called a laparoscopy, which is performed under general anaesthetic. A minute telescope is passed into the belly button to enable the surgeon to have a view of the outside of the uterus and the tubes. Coloured dye is then injected into the cervix, so the surgeon can observe if the tubes are functioning properly.

Treatment for tubal damage may involve surgery and, depending on the degree of damage, proceeding with IVF may be recommended.

Coping with investigations

Nobody enjoys invasive procedures, but it can be particularly difficult to undergo diagnostic procedures such as a laparoscopy. It is really important to get the mind on board: you want it working for you and not against you.

Think to yourself that this is a small part of the greater journey. By this stage in your fertility journey you need answers, and these answers will either point you on the right path or tell you there is nothing wrong. Either way, you are empowering yourself with knowledge.

Try not to pre-empt what the tests might find or let your imagination run away with you. It is much better to take it stage by stage. There is no point worrying about what might happen before it happens. Spend time preparing mentally before any procedure and try and paint a positive mental image. The mind is strong and can influence every cell in the body – so make your thoughts healthy and fertile, and try not to give into despair and lack of hope.

Affirmations
- Say these morning and night:
- 'I am strong and this knowledge will empower me.'
- 'I am fit and well and fertile.'
- 'I trust these professionals to do an excellent job – they have my best interests at heart.'

Underlying reproductive disorders

In women
Ovulatory problems
Ovulatory problems are the most common reason for women not to conceive. This is why I place such great emphasis on regulating your menstrual cycle and on visualizing the pro-

cess of ovulation. If you don't produce an egg in the mid-cycle then, obviously, there is nothing for the sperm to fertilize, and thus no conception.

If you are still having irregular periods after following my plan, or if you have any reason to suspect something is not right in this area, you should see your GP, who may refer you for tests. Please also see the box on the drug Clomid (page 284), which is given to help ovulation.

Irregular periods

As I have explained, problems with your period may indicate that you are not ovulating. If, however, you are having irregular periods, you can still conceive. I recommend that you follow my advice for your type in Part Two of this book, in conjunction with basal body temperature and checking your cervical secretions (see page 94), so that you know when in your cycle you are ovulating and you can have sexual intercourse during that time.

If you are still not getting pregnant, you may need to investigate whether you have polycystic ovary syndrome (PCOS), which is discussed below. This can be diagnosed by your GP.

No periods

An absence of periods is known as amenorrhoea. There are a number of factors that can cause your periods to stop completely, including:
- dramatic weight loss
- obesity
- stress
- emotional trauma
- frequent travel to different time zones
- an underactive thyroid (this may be accompanied by other symptoms such as fatigue, weight gain, fuzzy

thinking, low blood pressure, water retention – see *www. nhs.gov.uk* for more information).

If you have never had a period and you want to conceive, you need to contact your GP for tests straight away.

Polycystic ovarian syndrome (PCOS)

I have mentioned PCOS a number of times throughout the book because it is a common issue affecting fertility and one that is on the increase. As many as 20–33 per cent of women have polycystic ovaries, while between 5 and 10 per cent have PCOS.

PCOS is caused by a hormonal imbalance that causes the body to overstimulate the follicles in the ovaries. However, although a number of follicles begin developing, development is suspended before the follicle reaches the size it needs to be for ovulation to occur. The ovaries themselves are also over-sized. This can be seen on a scan. PCOS is usually diagnosed by ultrasound, but other methods include laparoscopy and blood tests. Symptoms of PCOS include:
- irregular periods or no periods
- being overweight and having difficulty in losing weight
- difficulty trying to conceive
- recurrent miscarriage[3]
- acne
- excess hair on the face or body
- mood swings.

From a Chinese medicine perspective, I see two variations of this condition in my clinic. First, there is the typical picture of PCOS, with weight gain due to Damp accumulation. In clinic we call this the 'Kidney Yang Deficient' type. The second comes out of a condition of Qi and Blood Deficiency. In clinic we call this the 'Kidney Yin Deficient' type.

As Jane Lyttleton, author of *Treatment for Infertility with*

Chinese Medicine explains: 'At one end of the PCOS spectrum there is the thin, wiry, restless, yin-deficient woman who ovulates irregularly or infrequently and has high testosterone, and at the other end is the overweight yang-deficient Damp woman, who may also have infrequent periods or have stopped ovulating altogether.'[4]

If you can easily identify yourself in either of these descriptions, it might well be worth following my plans for your type and seeing if your periods regulate and your condition improves at all.

You may already be working with a gynaecologist by now or be under the care of your GP. If you are working with an acupuncturist, I recommend that you discuss timing your acupuncture sessions around your mid-cycle to help with ovulation. You may have to pay close attention to your secretions (see page 94) and observe any breast or nipple tenderness in order to time this correctly.

Endometriosis

Endometriosis is another condition that I have mentioned a number of times so far. It occurs when the cells of the endometrium (the womb lining) start growing outside the uterus. The severity of endometriosis is determined on a sliding scale of stages one to four – and the level of pain you experience may not be indicative of the endometriosis you have. Some women only have a small amount and are in chronic pain, while others have it extensively, but feel nothing.

It is a common problem, occurring in roughly one in ten women of childbearing age, and it can cause infertility because of scarring, irritation and adhesion within the Fallopian tubes, preventing the smooth passage of the egg. It can cause damage to the ovaries and also implantation issues. Symptoms of endometriosis include:
• cramping pain in the lower abdomen, lower back, rectum

and even in the back of the legs
- severe period pain
- pain during intercourse
- painful bowel movements
- bleeding between periods
- heavy periods
- bloating
- pain on urinating.

Endometriosis is diagnosed by ultrasound or laparoscopy.

I urge those who know they have endometriosis to follow my advice for Blood Stagnation (see note on page 138) while working with a gynaecologist. The treatment you receive for endometriosis in Western medicine really depends on how badly you have it. In some cases, a gynaecologist will recommend laser surgery or diathermy to remove cysts and lesions. You may be treated with medicine in the form of oral pills, a nasal spray or an injection. The doctor may also suggest you take painkillers in conjunction with your medication.

Endometriosis can cause lasting damage to your reproductive organs, and even if it is cleared up you may still not be able to conceive naturally.

Q&A

My sisters both have endometriosis, does this mean I will also have it? It may mean you are susceptible to developing it. If you have a short menstrual cycle or experience painful periods or pain with sex you need to seek medical advice particularly if you are 30 or over and have not yet conceived.

Fibroids

These are firm lumps (benign tumours) that grow inside and outside the uterus – inside the muscle and under the lining. They can affect women of any age; as many as 40 per cent of women over thirty-five have them. Many women are not aware of them, but in a small percentage they cause problems, including issues with fertility. It's thought that they get in the way of the process by which the egg implants in the uterine lin-

THE ROLE OF BLOOD STAGNATION IN FIBROIDS AND ENDOMETRIOSIS

Bob Flaws and Honora Wolfe, both American practitioners of Chinese medicine, believe that modern-day issues, such as the use of the coil, terminations, the Pill, the use of antibiotics to treat venereal disease (which causes chronic Damp/Heat) and abdominal surgery, contribute to the rising numbers of women who are diagnosed with problems like endometriosis and fibroids. In their book *Prince Wen Hui's Cook*, they make the following dietary recommendations:

- **Avoid:** foods that aggravate the Liver (such as rich and fatty foods, red meat), eating late at night, alcohol and coffee.
- **Include:** aubergine, amasake, saffron, safflower, basil, brown sugar, chestnut.

However, they caution that: 'For treating long-standing Blood Stagnation, dietary modifications alone are seldom sufficient.' Where diet, acupuncture and herbs are not enough, Western surgery may be needed.

ing; they can also block the Fallopian tube and prevent the egg from being fertilized. Fibroids underneath the lining of the uterus may cause implantation issues. If they are near the entrance to the Fallopian tubes, they can cause blockages. Symptoms of fibroids include:

- abdominal pain
- heavy bleeding
- bleeding between periods
- anaemia
- pain during intercourse
- bloating
- urinary problems – in some cases the pressure from the fibroids on your bladder can make you need to go more often
- bowel problems – as above, the pressure can also cause constipation

- miscarriage and premature birth – fibroids can increase in size during pregnancy and create complications during birth.
  There may also be no symptoms at all.

Fibroids are diagnosed through routine examination or by pelvic ultrasound. There are a number of treatment options:

- Surgery – there is a range of surgical options, depending on your age and the severity of your fibroids. You need to discuss any surgery with your doctor as the procedure itself can cause scarring, which can contribute to fertility problems.
- Uterine artery embolization (sometimes referred to as UAE or UFE) – this procedure involves cutting off the blood supply to the fibroids. It has a 60–90 per cent success rate.
- Hormone treatments can shrink the fibroids, but are not suitable if you are trying to conceive.

If your fibroids are not causing you pain or are not large, many doctors will advise that you leave them alone.

Premature menopause

Premature menopause, or premature ovulation failure (POF), is the diagnosis for women who stop ovulating before the age of forty (the normal age being around fifty-one). Most of these women start experiencing symptoms of the menopause alongside irregular periods and less bleeding, but in some cases periods just stop.

Heavy smoking can accelerate the menopause, as can viral infections of the ovaries, but, in most cases, premature menopause runs in families and can be a side effect of hyperthyroidism (see below) and lupus. In rare cases the ovaries start working again on their own.

WHY AM I NOT GETTING PREGNANT?'

Symptoms of premature menopause include:
- irregular periods
- less bleeding or heavier bleeding
- long gaps with no menstruation at all
- hot flushes
- mood swings
- lack of vaginal fluid
- dry skin, eyes or mouth
- decreased interest in sex
- incontinence (lack of bladder control).

Diagnosis is with a blood test to determine FSH levels – a result above 30 would usually indicate premature menopause. Your doctor may prescribe hormone replacement therapy (HRT) to guard against osteoporosis; however, if you want to conceive you will need to explore the option of egg donation and IVF.

Immune system problems or immunologic infertility

It's thought that 20 per cent of 'unexplained infertility' could be the result of immune system problems where the immune system of the mother attacks or rejects the embryo.

Women prone to fertility problems have been found to have a significantly higher incidence of abnormal blood factors called autoimmune antibodies. In studies, women with abnormal autoimmune antibodies were 80 per cent less likely to conceive than those without and the presence of the autoimmune antibodies was found in the fluid that bathes eggs in the ovaries.

Such antibodies can cause both failure to conceive and repeated pregnancy loss (miscarriage), sometimes before a woman even knows she is pregnant. It also causes recurrent IVF or ICSI failure.

This is an area of focused research; for more information

see *www.argc.co.uk.* or *www.haveababy.com.*

To diagnose, a blood test will be performed to check for antibodies. Antiphospholipid antibodies are thought to be a common cause of recurrent miscarriage, especially first-trimester miscarriage. Other antibodies that have been identified are thyroid antibodies, anti-nuclear antibodies and lupus antibodies. It is also thought that abnormal NK (natural killer) cells can also play a role.

Some private IVF clinics may treat elevated NK cells by giving an IVIg infusion – an intravenous drug that helps suppress the immune system.

Note: if you are diagnosed with NK cells, it is important to have your thyroid monitored. Approximately 5 per cent of women with elevated NK cells go on to develop hypothyroidism.

Thyroid

Although fairly common, thyroid disorders are often overlooked, undiagnosed or poorly treated. Many women suffer from thyroid dysfunction which can prevent pregnancy from occurring, particularly in the case of hypothyroidism (underactive thyroid). The presence of thyroid antibodies may also alert your doctor to a potential problem with conceiving.

One of the problems in identifying thyroid problems is that the symptoms differ from person to person. Some of the commonly reported symptoms are:

- exhaustion
- weight gain
- dryness of hair, nails and skin
- loss of libido
- sensitivity to cold and difficulty warming up
- mood changes
- constipation
- poor memory

- lack of concentration
- menstrual disturbances
- PMS.

I have observed that people diagnosed with thyroid problems are often very sensitive to stress and their environment. It is not clear whether this is the reason for their thyroid issue or a result of it, but I often make the following suggestions:

- Limit your exposure to chemicals: chlorine, plastics, fluoride (see the section on chemical quota, page 44 – this really applies to you).
- Drink bottled water, but from glass bottles only.
- Consider whether you may be allergic to any foods. Wheat can be a problem for some people; and wine can cause problems for sensitive immune systems because of the sulphates.
- Limit your exposure to things you are allergic to: if you are allergic to cats it's probably a good idea not to live with one. Being exposed to allergens can act as a low-grade irritant to the immune system, adding to the problem.
- Think about your digestion – how good is it? This is important, as a weak or leaky gut may interfere with absorption.
- Be aware of parasites. This is a bigger problems than you might imagine. Parasites living in the body can disrupt the delicate eco-system and aggravate autoimmune problems.
- Watch your stress levels. Stress can set off autoimmune problems, and thyroid problems often develop after periods of stress. Childbirth is a common trigger.
- Limit your time with people who are negative or who complain a lot and who generally 'leach' your energy.
- Use acupuncture.

- Improve relaxation and reduce stress through meditation and affirmations.

Miscarriage

Miscarriage is often not taken particularly seriously in Western medicine, unless it results in complications. Many women go straight back into work, sometimes the following day. Chinese medicine has a different view and considers the experience to be as draining as childbirth. And there is also the emotional impact of a miscarriage to consider, particularly when the pregnancy has taken a long time to conceive or was a result of IVF.

About half of all fertilized embryos never implant or do not implant sufficiently to become a pregnancy. Sometimes a woman may sense that she was briefly pregnant or may even get a faint positive early pregnancy test, but it then fails to progress.

Most miscarriages happen in the first trimester (95 per cent) and 15 per cent of all pregnancies will end in miscarriage. Lesley Regan states that 'A quarter of all women who become pregnant will experience at least one miscarriage – it is the most common complication of pregnancy.'[5]

Reasons for miscarriage

- Genetic – an embryo is the result of a successful union between sperm and egg and the genetic make-up of the egg is a result of both these factors. It is thought that up to 50 per cent of pregnancies fail due to chromosomal abnormalities, and the chances of this increase with age (in both sexes).
- Hormonal – progesterone produced by the corpus luteum supports the pregnancy in the first few weeks until the

placenta is fully established and so if you are deficient in progesterone this can cause miscarriage
- Blood-clotting disorders may play a role in approximately 15 per cent of all miscarriages
- Common vaginal infections such as bacterial vaginosis (BV)
- Structural problems with the cervix and uterus. These include: uterine fibroids, uterine scarring, a heart-shaped (bicornuate or double) uterus, a uterine septum (band of tissue running down the middle of the uterus) or an incompetent cervix (where the cervix does not remain closed, resulting in miscarriage after fourteen weeks; the treatment for this is a surgical stitch at twelve weeks).
- Autoimmune antibodies.
- Unknown causes.

Whatever the cause of miscarriage, I believe that recovery and proper aftercare are vitally important in preventing a recurrence. Following a miscarriage, a woman needs time to collect herself and her feelings, and going straight back to work may not be the right thing. There are those who say, 'Well I just wanted to forget about it and move on – get on with my life.' I caution these women not to be too tough: I see so many who are haunted by miscarriage years later. I recommend the following:
- Give yourself some emotional and physical time out – your body is pumped full of pregnancy hormones and the drop in these will contribute to feelings of sadness. Your breasts may have grown and your abdomen may have swollen, which will make you feel as if you are still pregnant, even though you are not.
- Grieve – this is an important part of the process.
- Take your mind off it, but try to do this through pleasurable things, rather than throwing yourself into your work.

- Don't expect too much of yourself.

When to start trying again

This is a highly emotive question, and one that elicits a variety of answers from the medical community. Some obstetricians say it's OK to try in your next cycle; others say that you should wait for three cycles.

I think it very much depends on the nature of the miscarriage. If the miscarriage was due to a problem with the embryo, for example, or was very early on, then waiting may not be the best option. However, if the miscarriage was due to an infection, or it resulted in heavy blood loss, you would be well advised to wait a few months (four months is good, time permitting).

The body needs time to repair and get back into balance. The last thing you want is to go through the trauma of miscarriage again, so although the idea of falling pregnant as quickly as possible is very tempting, investing time in preparing the soil will pay off in the long run.

My approach

My recommendations for patients who have miscarried will vary according to the circumstances. It is worth mentioning that clinical trials demonstrate that women who receive support and continuity of care following a miscarriage go on to have successful pregnancies.[6]

- If a patient has a history of miscarriage, I will spend time correcting any energetic imbalances and advise following the pre-conception plan (Chapters 4–7) for at least four months.
- In the case of a threatened miscarriage, I will try to see if we can apply some treatment to save the pregnancy. Acupuncture, for example, will not save a pregnancy with a genetic abnormality, but in many other cases there

CASE STUDY: AN EXPERIENCE OF REPEAT MISCARRIAGE

My next birthday is my fortieth. I have been pregnant three times and each time lost my baby. I can feel the deep sense of grief welling up and pressing on my chest like a huge heavy hand as I write. My clock has been ticking with increasing intensity since my early thirties; sometimes it is so loud now that it completely takes over my being.

Finding out I was pregnant for the first time was such a joyful experience, full of innocent anticipation and the promise of motherhood. When the first spots of blood started, followed by cramping, I went completely into shock. I couldn't believe what was happening; it felt animalistic, an out-of-body experience. I was a helpless heap. I had to just let go. It was what it was.

The last pregnancy ended three months ago, I was twelve weeks pregnant and I thought surely this time it was meant to be. Yet at my three-month scan, my hormone levels were not right and I was advised to undergo a CVS (Chorionic Villus Sampling test). My baby died following the procedure.

I will never get over the loss that I feel from these events, the emptiness and pain that follows: they are part of me now. However, as they say, with deep suffering you start to glimpse your true nature. Good can come out of these times. I have learnt much about how to 'be', trying to flow with my emotions, and not to hang on to or hide the pain.

Since my first miscarriage, I have become an acupuncturist, a yoga teacher and now a herbalist too. I practise dealing in the detail of moments. In one moment I feel OK, in the next briefly happy, then grief or anger or even nothing. I try and focus on the small things during the day. By doing this, I am dealing in the now, not controlling my future or holding on to the past. I learnt to live in the moment – that has helped me. It continually reminds me that whatever is happening to me – a moment of joy or a moment of suffering – it is going to pass and turn into something new.

Annee, a great friend of mine, gave me the best piece of advice. She said, 'There is only so much you can do to make yourself baby ready: eat well, sleep well, use techniques to look after the self, then let go and leave the rest up to the universe. You can only control so much.' This is what I do, every day.

Today, the sun is shining outside, my dog is cutely growling and grumbling on the floor next to me, my heart feels a little heavy from writing this piece, but I feel positive. Who knows what tomorrow might bring? I could find out that I am pregnant again, and this time it could last. It is what it is.

may be some hope.

- After a miscarriage, it's important to be back in balance before attempting again. I recommend following my plan for four months for Blood Deficient, Blood Stagnant, Yin or Yang Deficient or Heat types. Those with other tendencies may be able to try a little sooner.
- Miscarriage can occur because the mother is very weak; in such cases, taking it really easy during the first trimester (i.e. the first twelve weeks) is very important.
- Blood Deficiency is a common cause of miscarriage in Chinese medicine; patients who are Blood Deficient need to make sure they follow the plan for it and rest, rest, rest.
- Heat – leading to Reckless Blood (see page 138), perhaps as a result of Yin Deficiency is also common. Heat types must ensure that their diet is bland with no spicy foods or heating substances. They should avoid coffee too. It is also important to keep a calm and cool mind. This condition would relate to infection in Western medicine.
- Blood Stagnation types have to be careful to avoid any physical trauma or bruising to the uterus. This condition includes the blood-clotting issues in Western medicine and would be treated with heparin or aspirin if blood-clotting factors are suspected. Patients who know they are prone to Blood Stagnation need to prepare really well prior to pregnancy.

Once you start trying to conceive again, the question 'Is the mind on board?' is more important than ever: you really need to keep a strong mental imagine of the pregnancy succeeding. So, spend time every day visualizing the pregnancy continuing. I suggest you do this for at least ten minutes, three times a day, to confirm the image in your mind's eye. It is vital to see what you wish to happen and to put your faith in it.

Negative mental dialogue is emotionally draining. If you find you are obsessing about miscarrying, try to reset the mental loop so that every time you start to worry, you repeat an affirmation instead:

- 'My body is strong and my mind is calm.'
- 'I am able to carry this pregnancy to term.'
- 'I have everything I need to carry a pregnancy to term.'
- 'I rejoice in my pregnant body and I am confident the pregnancy will continue.'

Secondary infertility

Secondary infertility is the inability to conceive or carry a pregnancy in a woman who has had a previous pregnancy. Many people do not see it as a fertility issue though – medical professionals are often less inclined to give treatment; while family and friends are not always sympathetic – which makes it very difficult for those who experience it. The problem is that many people, including doctors who don't specialize in this area, believe that once you have conceived you will be able to conceive again. It is not uncommon for couples to be sent away with the brush-off: 'Just keep trying.'

Secondary infertility is, however, a serious issue, accounting for as many as 60 per cent of fertility cases.

What causes secondary infertility?

The causes are the same as for any case of infertility.

For women, issues cited in secondary infertility include:

- problems ovulating
- endometriosis
- pelvic adhesions (which can be caused by Caesarean section, or other abdominal surgery, the coil or IUD, instrumental deliveries and post-partum haemorrhage).

Also, bear in mind that a woman with secondary infertility is older than when she last gave birth; she may also have gained weight, developed a less healthy and less active lifestyle and be working harder (being a mother is hard work too). And, as we have seen, small changes in health, lifestyle and outlook can affect reproductive health.

There's the emotion factor. My colleague Emma Roberts says: 'More often than not it is due, emotionally at least, to a trauma of some sort the first time round – possibly a traumatic birth, possibly postnatal depression or other experience, such as a lack of support from husband or the family. I also see women who are anxious that they will not cope – they are already struggling with one child.'

Emma uses hypnosis, affirmations and meridian tapping to help women release any anxieties that may be standing in the way of them conceiving again.

In men, the issues cited include abnormalities with sperm and problems ejaculating.

I think it is worth seeking medical advice, particularly if age is a significant factor (i.e. you are thirty-five or over).

Supporting men through infertility

It was not so long ago that infertility was considered a purely female issue. Thankfully, this is no longer the case and male infertility is now recognized as the cause in 30 per cent of cases and as a contributing factor in another 40–45 per cent. Historically, it has been easier for Western medicine to treat female infertility than it has been to address the problems caused by male infertility (this was certainly the case before ICSI) and it is often assumed that men need not be offered treatment. However, acupuncture has a long history of treating male infertility: in the short term it can improve libido and

CASE STUDY: SECONDARY INFERTILITY

Sophie was thirty-four years old and had conceived her first son within two months of trying, four years earlier. She had a straightforward pregnancy, but had lost a lot of blood shortly after labour. She found it difficult to cope in the early weeks, initially struggling to breastfeed. But she got there in the end and managed to keep it up for fourteen months.

When Sophie came to see me in the clinic, she looked worn out, with a dry appearance to her skin and hair. She explained that she and her husband had started trying to conceive their second child when she stopped breastfeeding. It was now two years down the line and nothing had happened – all her friends were pregnant again and she felt desperate and anxious.

I asked her when her periods had resumed and some details about the flow and quality of the blood. She told me that they were much lighter than they had been before she was pregnant. She also told me that emotionally she had changed too. These days, she felt quite anxious at times and was upset in this change in character – she had always been the life and soul of the party with bags of energy.

As some women do, Sophie had lost a lot of weight after the birth and was now lighter than she had been at any point in her life before. I suggested that she saw her GP to have her thyroid tested. From a Chinese medicine point of view, I felt she was Blood Deficient, but that there was also an issue with her Heart. I explained that the blood loss at birth, followed by the extended breastfeeding, had made her Blood Deficient. She had not quite caught up with the sleepless nights following in the birth of her son and this lack of sleep was adding to her anxiety.

Over the course of the treatment, Sophie's skin and hair quality improved. Her mood lifted too and she became less 'fixed' on achieving a pregnancy and more focused on regaining her own strength and energy. Her menstrual bleed became fuller and she enjoyed the quiet time she carved out for herself around her period.

Happily Sophie conceived on the fourth cycle of treatment and had a baby girl nine months later with no complications.

sperm motility, while three months of treatment can successfully treat sperm morphology, thereby improving the quality of the sperm.

Men can be overlooked in the fertility journey, sometimes because they don't want to be involved, but frequently because they are unaware of what is on offer. So, we need to get the men on board by encouraging them to:

- get tested
- adapt their diet and lifestyle to get healthy for conception
- try alternative therapy, such as acupuncture, aromatherapy and massage to help increase libido around ovulation for natural conception
- use acupuncture for issues of premature ejaculation and erectile dysfunction
- become involved in the IVF journey – in my experience, the cases where both partners are involved and where the man is treated, for example with acupuncture, show a higher rate of either successful first-time IVF or the woman falling pregnant naturally following IVF (within two menstrual cycles).

Tests for men
Questions the GP might ask you
General
- How old are you?
- How much do you weigh?
- Do you have any sexual problems – premature ejaculation, erectile dysfunction?
- How long you have been trying to conceive?
- How often do you have sex?
- Do you have undescended testicles?
- Do you take/have you taken any medication – such as cancer treatment?
- Have you had any serious illnesses?

- Have you had any operations in the genital area or for a hernia?
- Have you ever had mumps?
- Are you aware of any other medical issues?
- Is there any relevant family medical history?

Sexual history
- How many partners have you had?
- What contraceptives have you used?
- Have you had any sexually transmitted diseases?

Lifestyle
- Do you work with heat, for example as a chef?
- What are your working hours?
- What are your stress levels like?
- Do you smoke?
- How much alcohol do you drink?
- Do you take recreational drugs?
- What is your diet like?
- What exercise do you take (e.g. cycling)?
- Do you regularly take hot baths, wear tight briefs or Lycra while exercising?

What to expect from a basic examination
The GP will check a number of things that may include your BMI, blood pressure and general appearance to assess overall health and genitals (they may check for any pain, swelling or variation in size which may indicate undescended testicles). They will take a swab, if you are at risk of having an STD.

You may also be asked for a sperm sample, and it is important that you have not ejaculated for two or three days before the sample is produced. Your sperm will be tested for:
- motility (its ability to move)
- morphology (its shape – poor morphology indicates a

CASE STUDY: IRON MAN

Juliette (aged twenty-eight) and her partner, Archie (twenty-nine), had been trying for six months to conceive with no luck. They came directly to me, without seeing their GP or a gynaecologist.

I did the 360-degree check on both partners. Juliette had a slightly irregular cycle. Archie had not had a sperm test. I discussed with them how quickly they wanted to push things forward – did they want tests straight away or did they want to try my cycles first? Both were reluctant to go straight for tests and decided to do four months of my cycles first. We decided to revisit the testing question if they hadn't conceived after this.

After four months, they hadn't conceived, but were in markedly better health. Juliette's cycles had become regular – bang on twenty-eight days – and Archie was a lot less restless after reducing his intake of coffee, alcohol and other heating substances.

We decided that it wouldn't hurt to take the next step, so I suggested that they have some basic tests with their GP. Juliette went immediately and her tests revealed that her progesterone was low – this backed up my own findings that the luteal phase of her cycle was slightly deficient. Her GP prescribed progesterone suppositories and I advised her to continue seeing me twice a month, but only in the luteal phase (post-

ovulation), where we would do some warming-the-womb treatments.

Two cycles later, Juliette had still not conceived, despite a considerable improvement. At this stage, I considered there to be nothing significantly wrong with her and urged her to get her partner tested.

Archie finally agreed to have a sperm test. It showed a very high level of abnormal forms with only 2 per cent normal. This often indicates Heat in Chinese medicine. Archie admitted that he had found it hard to stop his Iron Man training which involved cycling, running and weight-lifting. He could not understand that it was unhealthy for him and pointed out that he had significantly reduced his intake of spicy foods and red wine (although he still had a regular curry night with the boys). All in all, he was generating quite a lot of Heat in his system, which can, in turn, damage sperm's morphology. Archie was horrified that such a seemingly 'healthy' existence had damaged his sperm, but it was the catalyst he needed to get on with the plan.

The couple took some time out from trying until Archie finished his Iron Man training, then after two months on the 'male cycle', they tried again. They conceived and baby Samuel was born in November 2008.

high level of abnormal sperm cells, e.g. two heads, no tails, etc.)
- sperm count
- volume of semen (seminal fluid carries the sperm cells);
- viscosity (thickness)
- white and red blood cell count (high levels of either may indicate infection)
- pH – to check it is not too acidic
- clumping – which can be a sign that the body is making anti-sperm antibodies.

Other tests
The male partner can take a blood test to determine sex hormone levels:
- Testosterone – low levels *may* indicate testicular failure according to obstetrician Michael Dooley, but may also be indicative of other issues.
- Follicle-stimulating hormone (FSH) – this is essential for sperm development. High levels can suggest testicular failure and problems with sperm production.
- Luteinizing hormone (LH) – high levels of LH and a low level of testosterone can indicate testicular failure. ICSI may be an option.
- Fructose test – this tests for obstructions in the seminal vesicles. If no fructose is found it is usually indicative of a blockage.

They may also have the following tests:
- An antisperm antibodies test – as with women, it is possible for a man's immune system to over-respond and kill off his own sperm as if it was a bacterial invader.
- A sperm DNA fragmentation index – this checks DNA fragmentation which can cause recurrent miscarriage because of chromosomal abnormalities. Antioxidant

supplements can help.
- Chromosome testing – to determine whether there is a genetic abnormality that accounts for a couple's fertility issue.

Is the mind on board?

Getting pregnant requires effort and the mind is a powerful tool at your disposal.

Are family and friends on board?

The most important message you need to get across to family and friends is: have compassion. The infertility journey is a difficult one and, with the best will in the world, friends and family can make things worse with comments, advice and questions.

Many of my patients tell me it would be great if there was something they could give people to read. Here it is:

Friends and family – what can *you* do?
- Listen – being a good listener is a skill for life. It is not easy and most people are not that good at it. The thing about listening is that you don't actually have to say a thing; in fact, that is really the point. You just connect with the person, and listen to what they are saying to you.
- Be sensitive: don't say things like, 'You really need to relax more,' or 'I just know you will be all right – I just feel it.' Or if someone has one child, don't tell them: 'Think of what you already have – you are lucky.'
- Give your time – this is a precious commodity. Turn your phone off and spend quality time with them.
- Don't give advice, unless it is specifically sought. Advice

can really be confusing. Infertility is a highly specialized field, and it's likely that the couple going through the process knows more than you do (unless of course you are a specialist!). You also run the risk of contradicting what a specialist may have told them and so create a conflict.

- Avoid the word 'should' – this is a big one. I try not to use it too – although it's sometimes easier said than done. It's often the case that we tell someone what they *should* be doing because they appear vulnerable and we think it's what they want to hear. However, it is very disempowering. A better way is to let them bounce ideas off you so that they can reach their own conclusions.
- Ask – don't tell. Simply say: 'What can I do to help you?'
- Support their choices: they may have agonized a great deal over making them, so try not to undermine them.
- Respect their right to privacy – don't dig for information if it is not offered.

And a note to you – the patient

Asking too many people for advice can be confusing: you need to find a balance between arming yourself with information from books, magazines and the specialist, and asking everyone around you for their opinion. It's also wise to avoid searching obsessively for answers on the Internet, which can sometimes be misleading. While information can be empowering, it can also add to stress.

My advice is to still your mind with yoga and meditation. Use your breath to calm your body. Listen to your intuition. Try to hear the clear voice within you, as well as the cacophony around you.

And finally, keep this ancient saying in mind (quoted by the Chinese medicine practitioner, Heiner Fruehauf in an article on emotions in Chinese medicine): 'Compassion is manifested by loving others, not by loving self; selflessness is manifested by straightening out the self, not by straightening out others.'[7]

Chapter Nine

The ART cycle – for those undergoing IUI, IVF and ICSI

You may have arrived at this point via any number of paths. Perhaps your test results brought you here, or maybe you've followed my advice through the cycles and you are now ready to move on to the next stage. Or you may have embarked on IVF before coming to this book. Either way, the decision to pursue Assisted Reproductive Technologies (or ART) is an enormous one, and I am here to support you through this next step and to offer tips and advice for optimizing your chances of conceiving this way.

I am also here to give you the Chinese medicine perspective; it is now widely accepted in the medical community that women who have acupuncture during IVF are 65 per cent more likely to go on to have a successful embryo transfer procedure and 91 per cent more likely to have a live birth.[1] And there are other supporting therapies and practices, such as meditation, yoga, meridian tapping and aromatherapy, which may also increase your chance of conceiving with ART. (Do let your specialist or clinic know that you are using this book and any other complementary and alternative medicine (CAM) in conjunction with your fertility medicine.)

Assisted conception can, at times, be a cold and clinical experience, a long way from the nurturing warmth we associate with the notion of fertility and motherhood. Equipped, however, with the skills and tools you have learnt thus far, you can counter all this with warmth, love, good health and positive thinking. I genuinely believe this will enhance your chances of conceiving.

Understandably, some patients lose sight of why they are here – with the focus so heavily trained on the details of conception, it's easy to forget the bigger picture. So, throughout all the procedures, keep in mind an image of yourself with your baby.

Some of you, especially those whose treatment is on the NHS, may have to wait before fertility treatment can start. Throughout this waiting time, continue doing the cycles (Chapters Four to Seven), and for as long as your particular case allows. And remember that sign in my office: 'Expect a miracle'. I've certainly seen a few; so, don't give up on yourself.

In this chapter, I am going to take you briefly through the different options that come under the umbrella term ART. I will give you an idea of what to expect – although procedure does vary from clinic to clinic – and ideas for questions you can ask.

I should add that I am not going to go into intricate detail on all the medical aspects of ART. You will be overloaded with information – consent forms, information packs, latest research figures, etc. – from your clinic. Plus, there are countless books devoted solely to this subject and you have probably already spent quite a lot of time reading around the subject on the Internet. Like most of my patients going through IVF, what you'll really want to know now is what *you* can do to enhance your chances of conceiving while using fertility medicine. And that's why I am here.

I will give you tips on how to stay healthy through the

process and how to get your mind on board (which is half the battle, as I always tell my patients). So, while you are in the clinic, be the patient; when you are out of the clinic, do everything you can for yourself.

What are Assisted Reproductive Technologies (ART)?

Assisted Reproductive Technologies are the use of medical intervention to achieve pregnancy, wholly or partially with medical assistance.

The use of such technologies continues to rise in the UK. In 2007, 36,648 women received fertility treatment – an increase of 5 per cent on the previous year. In 2006, 12,589 babies were born as a result of IVF and ICSI, an increase of nearly 12 per cent on the previous year. Forecasts suggest those figures will continue to rise in the near future. Today, more than twice as many women are having treatment as had it in 1992, according to the Human Fertilization and Embryology Authority (the HFEA).[2] For the purposes of this book, we will be discussing:

- clomid
- IUI (intrauterine insemination)
- IVF (in vitro fertilization)
- ICSI (intracytoplasmic sperm injection)
- donor cycles.

The time factor

Assisted conception needs some forward planning. The procedures, like the investigations, can take time to organize. I strongly urge you to sit down and setting out a plan of action with your doctor or fertility clinic. And be prepared for that plan to change.

For some couples, time is an issue and this means that assisted conception on the NHS is not an option. Others will not be eligible for treatment on the NHS (see below).

The money factor

The financial implications of being treated at a private clinic are considerable. Private medicine is expensive and, to date, you cannot receive treatment on private medical insurance (although some insurance will cover investigations and treatment for miscarriage).

To give you an idea, at the time of going to press, the cost of IVF can vary between £3,000 and £5,000 per treatment cycle, depending on which clinic you use. Treatment on the NHS is free, of course, but you need to be eligible and you may need to wait. The National Institute of Clinical Excellence (NICE) guidelines currently suggest that couples should be offered up to three cycles of IVF on the NHS if the woman is aged between twenty-three and thirty-nine. Local health authorities will apply their own eligibility criteria. (For more on NHS treatment, see *www.nhs.gov.uk*.)

You and your partner need to work out how much the entire treatment will cost you in advance – factoring in other considerations, such as time off work, travel costs, accommodation and so on.

Clomid/Clomifene

Clomid is a first-line fertility drug that is given to women with unexplained infertility or women who are not ovulating, and it can be prescribed by the GP.

Clomid stimulates ovulation and can be used alone or in conjunction with IUI. Research has shown, however, that unless a woman is unable to ovulate, the use of clomid on its own has questionable benefits. It certainly increases the chances of becoming pregnant with multiples.

Personally, I do not advocate the blanket use of clomid. Every drug has adverse effects and, in the absence of a justifiable reason, I think the natural approaches – such as acupuncture – are often more suitable. However, in the case of Kidney Yang deficiency – the Damp-type polycystic ovary syndrome (PCOS) I outlined in the last chapter – it does have benefits. It is classed in Chinese medicine as a 'hot' drug, and can really assist the release of an egg in a Damp and sluggish system.

I don't recommend clomid for Blood and Yin Deficient types. Typically, the follicles don't mature in these patients and their endometrium doesn't reach the required 8mm thickness for implantation to occur. It can also cause restlessness and anxiety. If you have already responded poorly to it, this may mean that you are Blood and Yin Deficient.

Where it is suitable, I recommend that you use clomid for a maximum of three months; after this, the side effects of the drug may kick in, including:

- drying up of fertile mucus
- irritability
- poor follicle development
- thinning of the endometrium
- blurred vision
- headaches
- weight gain
- pelvic pain
- abdominal pain
- swelling.

Tell your doctor if you experience any side effects.

Intrauterine Insemination (IUI)

IUI (which used to be called artificial insemination) involves the sperm being inserted directly into the uterus at ovulation to increase the chances of conception. The idea is that the sperm have a better chance of reaching the Fallopian tubes if injected using IUI. The clinic will scan you to pinpoint the exact time of ovulation. Many women are prescribed fertility drugs, such as clomid, at the same time.

Sometimes couples opt for IUI because it is a cheaper alternative to IVF.

When is IUI used?

IUI is used if there is an issue of:

- premature ejaculation
- impotence
- low sperm count, but otherwise healthy sperm
- slow-moving sperm
- donor sperm being used
- unexplained infertility

When is IUI not suitable?

IUI is not suitable in cases of:

- blocked Fallopian tubes
- increased numbers of abnormal sperm

IUI can be a great option because it is relatively straightforward and you can still follow the advice I have given you in Part Two for your menstrual cycle. Do take note of my cautions regarding clomid (above), however, and if you feel it isn't right for you, talk the options through with your GP.

What is the success rate of IUI?

The success rate for IUI is around 10–15 per cent, and that figure increases by around 5 per cent if you are also taking clomid.

As yet, we have no statistics for the success rates of those receiving acupuncture in conjunction with IUI, but from my own clinical experience, I would highly recommend it.

In Vitro Fertilization (IVF)

The birth of Louise Brown, the world's first 'test-tube baby', on 25 July 1978, marked a huge leap in medical science. Thirty years later, more than 12,500 IVF babies are born in the UK every year, and hundreds and thousands more worldwide.

IVF involves taking sperm cells from the male partner and retrieving eggs from the female partner and allowing fertilization to occur in a laboratory. The fertilized egg or embryo is then returned to the uterus to implant naturally. There are four basic stages to the procedure:

- You will be given hormone drugs that will stimulate your ovaries for 'superovulation', which means that your body will produce multiple follicles from which your eggs will be harvested.
- Those eggs are then collected. The number varies, depending on your age, but the clinic will want to avoid 'hyperstimulation' (see OHSS, page 304).
- The collected eggs are then mixed with your partner's sperm for fertilization to occur.
- A fertilized egg, now termed an embryo, is then transferred back into your uterus (or, if you are over forty, this may be two or even three), normally three days after harvesting.

You will then be given Progesterone to increase the chances of the embryo implanting. In some clinics you will also be given aspirin, heparin or steroids or Viagra to aid implantation.

When is IVF used?

IVF may be used:

- when the Fallopian tubes are blocked or damaged
- when one or both Fallopian tubes are absent or have been removed
- in women who have PCOS and do not ovulate
- when male infertility is a factor
- in conjunction with ICSI (see page 308)
- when donor eggs or sperm are being used
- for unexplained infertility.

What is the success rate of IVF?

Every year, around 35,000 women receive IVF treatment in the UK, and 23.1 per cent of treatments result in a live birth.[3] Obviously, the chances of becoming pregnant depend on a number of factors, most importantly age and the original cause of a couple's infertility (if it is known). Every year the HFEA releases up-to-date figures to show the success rate of IVF treatment; these are available on their website *www.hfea. gov.uk*.

Figures do vary slightly from clinic to clinic, and some couples prefer to research the options in terms of success rates and price before making a choice.

An overview of IVF

Long protocol

This refers to the longer version IVF in which the body is 'down regulated' i.e. your hormones are shut down.

Down regulation

Down regulation medication is called GnRH. These drugs put your body into a temporary menopausal state, which stops your body's natural cycle and hormones, and so prevents any eggs from being released early. These drugs are normally in the form of a nasal spray (although some clinics use injectable medication) and are taken for 10–14 days, at the end of which the patient will be given a scan to make sure they have down regulated (and to check the thickness of the endometrium) before moving on to the next phase of the IVF cycle. At the time of the scan a blood test to measure hormone levels will be given in order to determine whether stimulation drugs can be administered.

Stimulation phase

During the stimulation phase the aim is to stimulate the ovaries to produce multiple follicles from which eggs will be harvested. The stimulation drugs are always injected by the patient herself for a period of 10–14 days. The patient will be regularly given scans during the stimulation phase to track the growth of the follicles and to monitor for OHSS (see page 304).

Egg collection

After 10–14 days of stimulation drugs, the patient will administer a 'trigger' injection of HCG to ensure the final maturing of the eggs and the easy release of the eggs at collection. Thirty-six hours later the eggs will be collected.

The egg collection usually takes place under deep sedation (although clinics vary slightly on this). Whichever method is used

Q&A
Can I fly after embryo transfer?
There is no evidence that flying has any detrimental effect either on implantation or pregnancy. However, most of the panel agreed that it should be avoided, if possible, particularly when there has been a history of miscarriage. TIPS: if you must fly, try to wait seven days after transfer and, if the flight is longer than four hours, ask your GP or consultant about taking aspirin and/or heparin as there is an increased risk of DVT.

to sedate the patient, the egg collection process should be pain-free. The embryologist will mix the eggs with the sperm in order for fertilisation to take place. In some cases ICSI is required to achieve fertilisation (see page 308).

Embryo transfer

The patient is not sedated for this procedure. The transfer of successfully fertilised embryos will take place two, three or five days following egg collection. A five-day transfer is referred to as a blastocyst transfer and allows the embryologist to pick the strongest embryos. Bear in mind, not all embryos will develop into blastocysts.

One or two embryos will be transferred depending on your age and medical history. If there are any embryos remaining they will be considered for freezing.

After embryo transfer you will be given progesterone pessaries or a progesterone injection to support implantation. At this stage, it is important that you rest as much as possible (without taking to bed) until a pregnancy test is done about two weeks later.

Short protocol

The short or 'flare' protocol simply means that the period of time taking the down regulation drugs is omitted, from thereon it remains the same as the long protocol. The short protocol will start on day one of the menstrual cycle and is recommended in women who have previously responded poorly to stimulation or who have elevated FSH levels.

Occasionally clinics may opt to use the short protocol for other reasons which will be discussed with you.

Q&A

How many blastocysts should I transfer?
There are many factors to consider here: age, how long you've been trying, number of previous failed IVF cycles. However, there is currently a move towards single-embryo transfer and the HFEA now advises 'one at a time'.
TIPS: look on the HFEA website for the most up-to-date information on this. Ask yourself, do you want twins? Could you cope with twins? Can your body cope with a twin pregnancy? If the answer to any of these is 'No', I'd strongly suggest you only transfer one.

Natural IVF

In so-called natural IVF minimal or no medication is used and as a result you mainly produce one or two eggs per cycle. Some clinics are beginning to recommend natural IVF for older women as it is thought that a normal and thus viable egg is more likely to be recruited in a natural cycle.

The success rates are much lower (around 5–8 per cent), which means that some couples have to do several rounds to achieve the same success as IVF with drugs. The advantage is, of course, that you are not exposed to the IVF drugs.

Getting the best out of your IVF – before you start

So many patients ask me, 'What can *I* do?' Ideally, time allowing, I would like you to spend four months preparing with my baby-making plan following the specific advice for your type (see Part Two).

Many clinics will insist that your FSH levels are at a certain mark before allowing you to proceed with treatment. This can be heartbreaking when your levels are high, but there are still things you can do to get yourself back on track.

In her book *Women's bodies, Women's Wisdom: The Complete Guide to Women's Health and Wellbeing,* Dr Christiane Northrup says: 'Taking nourishment just for ourselves and not to please others is uncommon for women.' She says that women are too used to doing everything for others. 'Thinking with your heart takes practice, but if you faithfully learn to start thinking with your heart and pay attention to areas of your life that bring you joy and fulfilment, over time you will evoke biochemical changes in your body that will recharge your batteries.'

I really believe that my friend in the case study on page 294 fell pregnant because she sent a very strong message to her soul that this was the thing she most wanted. She had a

OTHER IVF TECHNIQUES

Assisted hatching
In order to successfully implant into the uterine lining, the embryo needs to hatch out of its protective protein layer (zona pellicuda) and attach to the walls of the uterus. However, sometimes the zona pellicuda may be too thick, or the embryo may not have enough energy to break through. In assisted hatching a small hole is made in the outer lining of the protective layer in an attempt to help the embryos hatch properly.

Oocyte vitrification
Historically, the only method for freezing oocytes (or unfertilized eggs) was a slow-freezing method; however, female eggs contain a lot of water. This makes freezing them more problematic, as when they are frozen, ice crystals can form within the egg and destroy the cell's structure. Vitrification is a specialized freezing technique whereby the egg is frozen very quickly. The speed of freezing means that ice crystals don't have time to form, thereby preserving the quality of the oocytes.

PGD
Preimplantation Genetic Diagnosis technology is offered to some patients. It is suitable for couples with infertility related to recurrent miscarriage or for those who have had repeated unsuccessful IVF cycles. It is also used for couples who are at risk of passing on inherited genetic disease to their offspring. The procedure can only be performed as part of an IVF cycle between egg collection and transfer whereby one or two cells are removed from each embryo through a procedure called embryo biopsy. The cells are then analyzed to determine which embryos are free of genetic abnormalities and therefore the most viable for transfer.

Immune screening
Some private clinics are beginning to look at immunological issues as a reason for pregnancy failure. Blood tests are performed in order to measure the status of the immunological environment within a woman's reproductive system. It is thought that an environment that is immunologically hostile may prevent implantation of an embryo resulting in no pregnancy or early pregnancy failure.

This area of fertility treatment is still new and there needs to be more research done in the area. The treatments used are often controversial and there are many different approaches to both diagnosis and treatment. All this can make for a very confusing time for the patient who may be given conflicting advice. Having said that, it is an interesting area of fertility treatment and one to watch. It is worth noting that treatments are often invasive and costly, and all these aspects need to be factored into any decision regarding treatment.

moment of pure clarity, realizing that she really needed to make these changes in her life, and she went for it.

In my experience, there is a window of opportunity in some patients where they can make a difference; they can improve things enough for a pregnancy to occur:

- Make lifestyle changes – it is important to nourish yourself on all levels. My friend did this by eating regularly, sleeping better, worrying less and doing something she loved. She put her health and her fertility first, instead of work commitments and other people's demands. Some people are able to make these changes and shift their perspective while remaining in a situation, while others need to remove themselves in order to make a difference.
- Cut out alcohol, smoking and coffee and eat according to your type.
- See my recipe for sauerkraut (cabbage is great for helping the hormonal changes in your liver), page 61.
- Use acupuncture to help bring down FSH levels (this is also recommended by some fertility clinics).

Preparation for those who haven't already done the baby-making plan pre-conception cycles

If you are about to start IVF or IUI, but you don't have four months to spare, there is still plenty you can do to optimize your treatment. In the weeks immediately before treatment, think in terms of nourishing your Blood and building your Qi reserves.

- Rest.
- Give up drinking alcohol and quit smoking.
- The yoga fertility sequence outlined in the Appendix really helps in the preparation stage.
- The qigong exercise on page 325 (called 'palm healing') is ideal preparation too. Both yoga and qigong are

designed to cultivate Qi rather than exhaust it. They will also help to calm the mind.

- Make sure you are well rested and calm and that you don't have too much stress around you. This is not the time to build a new extension, for example, or to have a taxing relative to stay. Keep it simple.

CASE STUDY: LOWERING FSH LEVELS

Receiving the news that you have high FSH levels can be very distressing, but it can also act as a wake-up call. One of my patients, who happens to be a friend too, worked in the fashion industry for many years. She worked long hours and travelled frequently. She took few breaks and, most of the time, ate standing up in a short break around mid-afternoon.

She came to me for help with period pain and, at that time, was not thinking about getting pregnant: she was twenty-eight. I picked up something on her pulse that concerned me about her fertility and asked her when she was thinking about having children. She brushed the question aside and I didn't press her, but in due course she came back to me to ask what my concerns had been. I suggested that she have an FSH test, because I felt there might be an issue.

She did. Her FSH level was eighteen, potentially indicating poor ovarian reserve and/or ovarian function.

My friend was devastated. She was twenty-eight and staring infertility in the face before she'd even considered the possibility of children. She took a long, hard look at her life and decided she would take some time out from work. Her focus would be to spend some time doing what she wanted to do for a while.

She really addressed her health and stress levels. We drew up a fertility plan, she came for regular acupuncture and followed the plan to the letter. For her 'Is the mind on board?' work she took up a voluntary position to learn gardening, determined to acquire a new 'fertile' skill. Actually, she suggested this without any prompt from me, but I saw it as a very appropriate form of exercise. She fell pregnant naturally after six months.

Although this is not backed up by clinical trials, I believe that FSH levels can be affected by your lifestyle and high stress and other issues do impact on your reproductive system. My friend managed almost to halve her FSH levels to ten.

- Be organized: make sure you have lots of Blood-nourishing foods in the larder (see store cupboard suggestions, below). Everyone needs a good blood supply during IVF and protein is very important. If you organize everything in advance, you will considerably reduce the stress on yourself during treatment.

Prepare mentally. Try to use the methods I have taught you throughout the book to keep the mind on board. Try to avoid the obstacles thrown in your way, and keep your stride. In Chinese medicine we call this state of being 'the free and easy wanderer'. You may not feel very free and easy, but working on this will help you move around any obstacles easily and skilfully.

If you have had raised FSH levels, you can work on affirmations and Emma Robert's meridian tapping (see page 318) to bring them down. Imagine them at the level you want them to be – set that in stone and don't allow yourself to think of them at any other level. Be positive – you can move mountains. And repeat, repeat, repeat.

IVF store cupboard

If you have already done my pre-conception cycles you'll be aware of the importance of nutritional preparation. You can still be mindful of your type here, but now that we are dealing with IVF and the drugs and procedures that involves, the general rule is to include lots of seasonal Qi- and Blood-nourishing foods:

- All green foods are helpful to support the Liver function.
- Dandelion tea: good for a congested liver; also improves digestion.
- Nettle tea for the blood.
- Green tea: contains catechins, which help protect the liver.

- Essential fatty acids: eating oily fish is also good for the liver.
- Nuts and seeds – great for snacks, as they are high in protein and they are good fats.
- Beans, soya, lentil, etc. – all these are high in protein.
- Tofu.
- A good supply of chicken stock – homemade if possible (see page 50). You can prepare it beforehand and freeze it.
- Chlorella, spirulina, Omega 3 and folic acid supplements and whey protein.
- Oily fish, such as mackerel.
- Plenty of leafy green vegetables.
- You will need to drink plenty of water while undergoing IVF, but try to avoid plastic bottles. Buy glass ones or use filtered water.
- Try to buy in bulk so that you don't have too much to think about while you are going through the cycle.
- Ginger is a perfect Yang tonic as it aids digestion, settles the stomach, reduces nausea, boosts energy and soothes premenstrual cramps.

Getting the best out of your IVF – during the cycle

Long protocol

Our aim in this phase is to avoid getting too overheated. The IVF drugs tend be rather 'hot' in Chinese medicine terms, and this can impact on the free movement of the Qi.

If you are doing a 'long protocol', I recommend you continue with a daily yoga practice. This is because the 'down regulating' drugs can make the Qi stagnate. In my clinic, we use acupuncture to keep the Qi moving freely and to prevent the build-up of frustration. Exercise is a great way to help this. If you find the full yoga sequence daunting, break it down somewhat. The 'palm-healing' qigong exercises (see page 325) are also brilliant. From this point on, follow the advice below for the short protocol.

Short or 'flare' protocol

If you are doing a 'short' or 'flare' protocol then you need to make sure the blood flow is going straight to your abdomen, so if you usually run or go to the gym, take a break from that now.

Yoga and qigong are much gentler, but only do the practice if you feel up to it. In your case, I want you to concentrate all your mental efforts on growing follicles. You are going to ask your body to perform something beyond what it would do if left to its own devices.

You may feel as if you are looking down a track punctuated with hurdles, and I agree this is a daunting proposition. But remember my advice: take one step at a time. Keep in mind the way that Joe Simpson faced his extraordinary journey in *Touching the Void* (see page 21). To concentrate on your 'journey' as a whole may be too distracting and draining, so focus instead on what you can achieve each day. You can use my ritual (see page 299).

I often ask my patients: 'How many follicles do you want to produce?' When they give me their answer I tell them: 'Ask yourself for that number. Visualize that number. And keep repeating that number.'

ACUPUNCTURE DURING IVF

As I've mentioned before, the BMJ recently published an article that collated results of several studies showing that women who had acupuncture were 65 per cent more likely to go on to have a successful embryo transfer procedure and 91 per cent more likely to have a live birth.[4] If you decide to go ahead and have acupuncture, tell your IVF clinic that you are receiving acupuncture.

Acupuncture as a preparation for IVF is as important as having acupuncture throughout the IVF cycle. You will have better general health and studies show you are more likely to carry a pregnancy to term. Acupuncture can also be used during the stimulation stage to even up the follicle growth. On many occasions, I have managed to stimulate a rather sleepy ovary to produce follicles, sometimes doubling the amount available for collection.

As more and more trials take place, with encouraging results, I hope that in the future acupuncture will be an optional part of the IVF procedure and that increasing numbers of clinics will adopt it. It should be administered by a trained acupuncturist and practised in the traditional way.

It's good to be focused on your intention. I also have some tips for diet:

- Eat lots of protein. Plant protein is preferable, as it's easier on the liver. According to Dr Fedon Alexander Lindberg, in his book *The Greek Doctor's Diet*, the best sources of non-animal protein are: nuts and seeds, beans, lentils, chickpeas (houmous), tofu and spirulina (this is an algae). He says, 'Vegetarians should eat onions and garlic with their proteins as these contain sulphurous amino acids that are also among our most important antioxidants.'[5]
- Chlorella and Super Greens – available from health food shops – are good, as are lots of leafy green vegetables, sprinkled with sesame seeds.
- Some IVF units make you drink lots of milk, in order to ensure that you get sufficient protein. This is not ideal for Damp types, but it's not for long.
- The 'stimulation' phase – which usually takes ten to fourteen days – is a good time for acupuncture. I think it's an idea for your partner to have acupuncture treatments too. Perhaps he could also follow the plan for his type. Most men have little involvement in the IVF cycle and it can be a great way to bring them in.

For everyone: the rituals

Rituals are a natural distraction technique for people under pressure and they play an important role in helping people feel calm and secure in times when they might otherwise be stressed. Affirmations, meditation and yoga practice are examples of rituals that can help steady us in tough times. They have a far-reaching impact on both body and mind.

You may find it helpful to have a routine of your own to help smooth the path of the IVF process. Below I have drawn up a suggested ritual that you can use during the stimulation phase of your IVF, but you can also devise your own, if you prefer. The important thing is that you include things that make you feel good and calm. And remember our 360-degree approach: Is the engine working? Is the fuel good? Is the mind on board?

Suggested daily ritual

- **Hot water and lemon** When you wake up, have a glass of hot water with half a lemon squeezed in to help your liver, which has a big job ahead.
- **Yoga and qigong** Spend ten to fifteen minutes doing some very gentle yoga or the qigong palm-healing exercise (see page 325).
- **Supplements** Take your chlorella or spirulina and any EPA (Bio-Oil is a good one) and folic acid supplements. Royal jelly is also good Qi tonic.
- **Breakfast** Eat a warming breakfast, perhaps porridge (oats or millet), with some chopped dried dates for sweetness. It's fine to have sweetness in your diet – but keep it at the start of the day. Your breakfast is just the right thing to help follicles grow. Go to town with ideas, make it fun – your heart will appreciate the lightness and fun.
- **Visualization** Focus on what you are trying to achieve at this point in the IVF cycle: during stimulation you are visualizing your follicles growing evenly and being nourished by a good blood flow. Think of your endometrium gradually plumping up like a soft velvet cushion. You can also imagine that the energy you have

Assisted Reproduction Technologies and Herbs

I am not a herbalist, but I do work with some extremely talented and safe herbalists who make a huge difference to my patients. If you have been using herbal medicine up until now as preparation to IVF, you will want to discuss with your clinic and herbalist if and when to stop using it. There are some instances when it could be beneficial, for instance around implantation, but most clinics will want you to stop using it while taking the IVF drugs. This is because there is little research on the drug/herb interactions and since both herbs and IVF drugs are powerful substances all parties will want to be as safe as possible.

produced through your palm healing (page 325) will
plump up the follicles even more.

- **Mid-morning protein drink** Make this for yourself from:
25g whey protein (Solgar is a good one or any powder
you can buy from health-food shops), 8 fl oz Rice Dream
(milk alternative) or rice protein (Biotics), a handful
of almonds or a spoonful of nut butter, a handful of
oats, a teaspoon of EPA (such as Biotics Bio-Oil) and
a few frozen berries, defrosted. (You could also add
some organic milled flax seed for bulk and to help your
bowels!) Whiz all the ingredients together in a liquidizer,
and there you have it. If you can't do this at work, do
it in the morning and take it with you. And if you can't
manage this at all, just make sure you do have a healthy
snack to keep you going. (Or try my friend Danielle

Warm & Spicy Rice Pudding

Serves 2 (or 1 ample serving)
(Not for Damp types)
600ml milk
3 cloves
1 teaspoon ground ginger
½ teaspoon ground cardamom
¼ teaspoon ground cinnamon
4 level tablespoons maple syrup, agave syrup or sugar
8 generous tablespoons Arborio risotto rice

Heat the milk over a high heat, then stir in all the other ingredients. When the mixture begins to boil, immediately lower the heat to the minimum, give it a stir and put the lid on. Keep an eye on it for the next 20 minutes (or until the rice is cooked according to the packet instructions), stirring every now and then to make sure the rice isn't sticking or clumping. After this time, it should look like rice pudding. Turn off the heat and let it sit for another 20 minutes, then remove the cloves and serve.

(This rice pudding is delicious in hot weather after being chilled in the fridge for a couple of hours too.)

Margulies' great rice pudding recipe – see page 300).
Remember, you are going to need a lot of strength to
grow those follicles.

- **Lunch** Have a good lunch; if you are at work then you
  will need to be organized. Your lunch needs 'warmth' to
  it so it shouldn't be all salad. If you fancy a salad that's
  fine, but have a warmish soup with it. Make sure that
  your salad has seeds and sprouts on it. (Note: watercress
  and beetroot are excellent for the blood; also, don't
  eat fruit for a good few hours after a main meal, as it
  ferments in the stomach and slows down the digestive
  process.)

- **Teas** Drink nettle tea throughout the day to help nourish
  your blood. And lots of room-temperature water
  (preferably between meals).

- **Lunchtime stroll** After lunch try to get out for a stroll;
  if you have a green space near you then go and be with
  nature – research show it's good for your health and
  helps to declutter your thoughts.[6]

- **Visualization** While you walk, use the time to connect
  back with your follicles and see how they are doing; put
  your hand on your tummy to check it is warm. Try to
  visualize for ten minutes if you can.

- **Late afternoon soup** After work or in the late afternoon
  have a small bowl of soup, made using your chicken
  stock (or vegetable for vegetarians) – chop up a whole
  pointy cabbage and a carrot and make a hearty cabbage
  soup. Your Liver will love the cabbage; your Blood will
  love the stock.

- **Evening relaxation** Banish negative or heavy thoughts
  and practise some positive thinking. Remember how
  important it is to keep focused and to be optimistic.
  Practise your favourite mind exercises – meridian
  tapping, visualization, affirmations. The more the merrier

(see page 318). Watch some TV for light entertainment, try reading something easy that amuses you or chat to friends – but don't get dragged into anything negative.

- **Supper** – Don't eat too late (7 p.m. is a good time, if you can). Eat something nourishing, e.g. sardines or mackerel, sweet potato, leafy green vegetables.
- **Bath time** – Have a nice, relaxing bath with a few drops of grapefruit essential oil, which is good for the Liver.
- **Meditation** – Dim the lights and practise the meditation techniques described on page 76.
- **Bed** – Try to get to bed by 10 p.m. Remember the restorative value of sleep (see Chapter One).
- **Affirmation** – Before you sleep, try a little affirmation, such as: 'Every day in every way it's getting better and better.' Or anything that makes you feel at peace.
- **Sleep** Try falling asleep to the self-hypnosis tape I described in Chapter One, page 77.

Getting the best out of your IVF – egg collection

This stage is all about helping to calm the body prior to transfer – which is when the maturing embryos are put back into the uterus.

I suggest that you spend ten minutes, three times a day, visualizing your embryos' cells dividing and subdividing, growing bigger each day. This can feel a little strange as the embryos are not currently inside you, but many of my patients find it helpful: one said she felt the mental bond as if it was a physical one, so that when they were transferred back it felt as if they had never really left her; another described visualizing her embryos growing together and helping each other along. She imagined that they were all 'buddies' looking out for each other. This, too, helped with the feelings of separation that so many women feel.

Poached Salmon Terrine

Serves 8
600g poached salmon, skin removed
400g Ricotta cheese
juice of ½ lemon
Maldon salt and black pepper
200g watercress

1. Flake the salmon by hand into a large bowl. Measure out approximately 400g of the salmon and mix it, by hand, with the ricotta and lemon juice, adding salt and pepper to taste, this should have a fairly smooth consistency.

2. Roughly chop the watercress.

3. Line a loaf tin with cling film leaving plenty of excess at the edges.

4. Layer the salmon and ricotta mix alternately with the flaked salmon, then the watercress in the prepared tin. There should be enough for two layers of watercress salmon flakes and three of the salmon and ricotta mix. Make sure you finish with a layer of salmon and ricotta.

5. Fold the edges of the cling film on to the top of the terrine and refrigerate for a few hours.

6. Before serving, turn the terrine out on to a dish and remove the cling film. Slice with a sharp knife and serve with a watercress garnish or a salad.

Pear & Ginger Tart

Serves 8
For the filling
8 pears   **1 x 350g jar stem**
100ml water   **ginger in syrup**
For the pastry
90g butter   **60g polenta**
115g plain flour   **2 egg yolks**
90g sugar

1. To make the filling, peel, core and quarter the pears and place them in a pan with the water and the syrup from the stem ginger jar, and 4 chunks of ginger. Simmer over a low heat until the pears are tender but not soggy.

2. Meanwhile, prepare the pastry. Blend the butter and sugar. Add the egg yolks, one at a time, blending well. Add the sifted flour and polenta and briefly mix. Wrap the pastry in cling film and leave in the fridge for 20 minutes.

3. Once chilled, roll the pastry out between two large pieces of baking parchment or cling film and use it to line a flan dish – you might find it easier to push the pastry into the edges with your fingers.

4. Sprinkle about a tablespoon of dry polenta on to the base of the tart and arrange the poached pears on top. Carefully spoon about 2 tablespoons of the pear syrup over the pears and bake in the oven at 180°C/350°F/gas mark 4 for about 30 minutes until lightly browned.

5. Boil the remaining syrup in order to reduce it a little and serve with the tart and some crème fraîche.

OVARIAN HYPERSTIMULATION SYNDROME (OHSS)

OHSS is a side effect of the stimulation drugs given during an IVF cycle and occurs in 1 per cent of cycles.[7] Fluid from the ovaries leaks into the abdomen causing bloating in all cases, mild, moderate or severe. The symptoms are:

- in mild cases – slight enlargement of the ovaries, abdominal pain and distension
- in moderate cases – pain, visible enlargement around the abdomen, nausea and sometimes vomiting, shortness of breath on exhalation
- in severe cases – severe pain on exhalation and shortness of breath.

Severe cases are rare (0.25 per cent). The majority of my patients who have OHSS have PCOS (see page 258). The condition usually occurs after ovulation and can worsen in pregnancy. In the case of a pregnant patient with OHSS, I use acupuncture for the delicate early weeks when the OHSS symptoms may threaten the pregnancy. Signs and symptoms to look out for:

- a dry mouth, which can mark the onset – I always tell my patients to be aware of an unusually strong thirst or dry mouth
- skin that is visibly Damp or Heat (if the skin is cool, there is more Damp and if Hot then Heat)

- fluid retention, which may lead to oedema
- a lack of urine
- abdominal distention
- dizziness
- stuffiness in the chest and/or shortness of breath
- loose stools with mucus

Tips to prevent OHSS include:
- drinking water
- eating a high-protein diet, to help metabolize the IVF drugs
- acting quickly – the quicker you catch this condition, the more chance you have of improving it.
- If you are concerned call your clinic's twenty-four-hour helpline or go to your nearest hospital A&E department. If you can, get acupuncture every day until symptoms subside. In my clinic, I arrange for patients to come daily on a significantly reduced fee in order to manage this condition. I find acupuncture prior to transfer particularly useful in women who are experiencing even mild OHSS symptoms.

Here I recommend that you follow the recommendations for the final menstrual phase (Chapter Seven). From now on, it is all about a warm womb and a calm mind.

Getting the best out of your IVF – embryo transfer

On the day of embryo transfer you are bound to feel nervous, but my advice is to relax as much as possible and think positively. Here are some additional tips for what to do on the day:

- Don't wear any perfume or perfumed creams. Embryos are very sensitive.
- Liver Qi Stagnation types need to work on relaxation techniques prior to transfer – if you are too tense it can make the process difficult.
- Imagine that you have prepared a beautiful and safe environment for your embryos to thrive. If you have followed the plan, the soil will be really healthy and receptive.

Practise affirmations:

- 'Everything is perfect. My embryos have everything they need to grow and thrive.'
- 'I am able to achieve and maintain a pregnancy.'
- 'I am happy and relaxed and everything has gone really well.'

Getting the best out of your IVF – after transfer

After transfer, my recommendations are as follows:

Q&A

Should I have total bed rest afterwards; if so, for how long? All agreed on this one – it is not necessary and may even increase the risk of DVT. TIPS: follow your instinct. Rest is very important for implantation and if you feel like lying down, do so. But don't take to your bed for long periods of time.

CASE STUDY: AN INTEGRATED APPROACH

Sophie, thirty-one, and George, twenty-six, had been trying to conceive for eighteen months. On the first consultation, Sophie came alone. Previous investigations from another specialist revealed that she had a mild case of polycystic ovaries – irregular and painful periods.

She had severe tubal damage and a laparoscopy to remove adhesions. With her right tube severely blocked and the left partially so, Sophie had been offered clomid to help regulate her cycle and induce ovulation.

George hadn't been offered tests. George worked in the building trade and Sophie worked as a secretary. She described their relationship as strong and loving. They both drank and smoked and occasionally used recreational drugs, and although Sophie had recently given up, George was reluctant to stop his party lifestyle.

Since Sophie's tubes were quite severely damaged, we decided that clomid was not our first-choice treatment and that before she took it or underwent any intervention, we needed George to have a semen analysis. We wanted the full picture.

George's tests came back and showed a low count and a high level of abnormal forms.

Sophie understood that she was likely to need IVF because of the Fallopian tube damage and the increased risk of ectopic pregnancy, but they were keen to take a more holistic/integrated approach. George now wanted to do as much as possible to improve his semen results. He was willing to address his lifestyle issues to help the situation.

On George's first acupuncture visit, as he lay down for his treatment, he took a mobile phone out of each of his pockets. I asked him how long he had been carrying them there; he said every day for about five years. I advised him to stop carrying the phones in his trouser pockets immediately.

After three and a half months' preparation, with regular acupuncture, nutritional therapy, hypnotherapy and meridian tapping, Sophie and George decided they were ready to attempt IVF. George had a semen analysis that showed his semen was now within the normal range and they were able to avoid ICSI. Both Sophie and George had acupuncture throughout the IVF cycle and Sophie also had an EFT session (emotional freedom technique, see Resources, page 357) after transfer.

They were successful first time and baby Grace was born in 2006. Both Sophie and George say that the process of making positive changes strengthened their relationship. George was looking forward to having a drink, but was glad to have kicked his smoking habit. He also said that he had enjoyed being able to be more involved in the process.

- Take it easy. This doesn't mean that you have to take to your bed for days, but take a few days off work if you possibly can. You have put your body through a lot and you want to give it the best chance now.
- Catch up with some little jobs around the house that you've been meaning to do for ages (but nothing too taxing).
- Don't take hot baths (and some clinics say no baths at all) because of the possible risk of infection or of overheating the Blood. Use the shower for a few weeks, and if you don't have one, try the old-fashioned 'strip wash' (wet flannel, soap and a basin of warm water).
- Be positive: don't be afraid to hope. Remember everything you have learnt about keeping the mind on board: 'What the mind conceives the body achieves.'
- Keep following all the implantation advice – mental and physical – that I suggested in Chapter Seven, and concentrate on keeping your lower abdomen warm, though not overheated.
- Don't have a strenuous social calendar: watch some comedy or funny movies. In Chinese medicine, laughter has direct benefits for our health and immune system.
- Go to bed early and if you can't sleep read something light and entertaining.
- And remember: 'Expect a miracle.' The world is full of miracle babies and there is every reason to believe you could have one too.

Q&A

Can I keep up my normal exercise, which includes running?
Opinions vary from no exercise to minimal. It seems to depend on who is doing it, what they are used to and how much they plan to do.
TIPS: follow the exercise plan outlined in this book to be completely safe, at the very least for two weeks following transfer. Slow down to a walk. After that if you are used to a high level of exercise and are missing it, reintroduce it slowly. Do not exercise to the point of sweating at any time you either are or might be pregnant.

Intracytoplasmic Sperm Injection (ICSI)

ICSI is the same process as IVF, except that after egg collection a single sperm is injected into the egg. It is mainly used in cases of low sperm count or high abnormal forms. It results in the fertilization of between 75 and 80 per cent of eggs if the sperm is viable.

When is ICSI used?

ICSI is used in the case of:

- low sperm motility (less than 35 per cent)
- poor sperm morphology
- a low sperm concentration
- IVF patients who had a previous cycle(s) with no fertilization
- IVF patients with a low rate of fertilization
- IVF patients who have a very low yield of eggs at retrieval (fewer than five to six eggs).

Some clinics only use ICSI for severe male-factor infertility, while some use it if you have undergone IVF with no (or low) fertilization. If you are uncomfortable with ICSI and you are a borderline case, you could ask your clinic if you can use half the eggs harvested for IVF and half for ICSI. Some patients prefer IVF because it allows the sperm to fertilize the egg naturally.

Anyone on the ICSI route should follow my advice in Part Two for their fertility type and also read the information on the IVF cycle (pages 287–291).

Egg donation

Egg donation is an option for women who are unable to produce their own eggs. This could be for any number of reasons including an absence of ovaries, ovarian cancer, women who are at risk of passing on a genetic disorder or because of premature menopause. It is also an option for women who are coming to motherhood later in life and whose own eggs are of poor quality.

I have seen many couples arrive at the place when egg donation becomes the most likely chance of them carrying a baby and becoming a parent. It is a difficult decision and not one to be taken lightly. However, actually making the decision to go for it can ease the stress. I always think that it is the information-gathering stage of any medical journey that can be the most stressful and painful. Once you have a plan in place, it gives you a focus and there will be lots to organize. I am not under-estimating the emotional rollercoaster you would have been on to get to this point, but I would like to point out some of the benefits.

Some eggs for egg donation are available through egg-sharing schemes run through IVF clinics. This is offered to re-duce costs. Good candidates for donating their eggs in this way are women who are having IVF due to male-factor infertility.

Generally speaking, the embryos used in egg donation will probably have come from a younger woman (but not always). Your partner's sperm will be used to fertil-

RISKS ASSOCIATED WITH IVF AND ICSI

One common concern is that babies born as a result of ART have a slightly higher risk of congenital defects (2.6 per cent as opposed to 2 per cent in natural conception). Talk to your clinic about these risks if you are concerned, and for more information contact the HFEA (see Resources).

Other risks are:

- An increased chance of conceiving multiples (twins, triplets or more).[8] Multiples carry greater risks of complications than single pregnancies.
- Drug reactions – some women have a mild reaction (headaches or nausea) to fertility drugs. There is also the risk of ovarian hyper-stimulation syndrome (OHSS) – see page 304.
- Ectopic pregnancy – there is a slightly increased risk that the embryo will develop in the Fallopian tube rather than in the womb; however, the risk is still very small and also exists in natural conception.
- There may be an increased risk of miscarriage in ICSI due to the integrity of the sperm.
- A male born as a result of ICSI may inherit his father's infertility.

ize the egg. Most of the egg donation I have experienced has been done in Spain where the donors do tend to be in their twenties. This has obvious advantages, in that the genetic integrity of the embryos is likely to be better than that of an older woman. In Chinese medicine theory this would improve the chances of the child being born with strong Jing.

In Chinese medicine it is thought that your soul enters you

CASE STUDY: FERTILITY TO MENOPAUSE

Jackie came to me for acupuncture with a referral from her consultant gynaecologist. She was thirty-nine and had been having irregular periods for a year; when she split from her husband she'd stopped altogether for six months.

Jackie understood that the stress of the break-up and its timing was significant (we talked about the link between the Heart and the Womb too). She was also hoping to have a pregnancy soon and initially went to the consultant regarding egg freezing. Her blood tests revealed hormone levels, particularly a very high FSH indicating menopause. Her mother had gone through her menopause at the age of forty.

This was devastating news. I persuaded Jackie to continue her integrated treatment, and she had regular acupuncture to reduce her stress and to see if her cycle could be regulated and her periods might return. The gynaecologist asked her to hold off having another blood test until the onset of a bleed, in order to get a true hormone reading.

After two months Jackie had a light bleed, but her FSH levels were still very high. She continued with acupuncture and Chinese herbs for another four months. There was no bleed and a further blood test revealed only slight changes.

During the course of treatment, Jackie had moved through a phase of life that came upon her unexpectedly. She allowed feelings of frustration and disappointment to surface, she accepted how things were and became hopeful of becoming a mother in another way.

Fertility journeys do not always bring you to the place you first hoped. Sometimes joy comes from an unexpected source, and it's always worth being prepared to re-evaluate your journey. Jackie is now the proud mother of twins born after egg donation.

during birth. This means that a baby born as a result of egg donation is considered a part of the birth mother who gives it its soul. This is the mother who gives birth to it. When the baby is born it lets out a cry from deep in its lung – this is the outward manifestation of the energy imparted from its mother.

In the UK, around 500 babies are born a year as a result of egg donation. As with sperm donation, if you choose to try for egg donation you need to consider all the implications in advance. By law, your clinic must offer you professional counselling. I have had many patients who have conceived through egg donation and some of them elected to keep this decision between themselves and their partner and not to tell family and friends. It is a very personal decision.

The donor's profile will be matched as far as possible to your own, in terms of your colouring, race and overall appearance. The donor is screened for disease. The eggs are not frozen and can be fertilized either using IVF or ICSI. Embryos that are not used, however, can be frozen and are often used later by couples who want their children to be full genetic siblings.

After they've reached the age of eighteen, children born as a result of donated eggs or sperm can contact the HFEA to find out whether they are related to the person they intend to marry or to simply get details of the donor.

Sperm donation

In the UK, around 2,000 babies are born a year as a result of sperm donation. This may be an option for you if your partner is infertile, if he has had a vasectomy or a failed vasectomy reversal. It is also an option for lesbian couples and for those who do not have a partner but who would like to have a baby.

The donor is screened for infectious diseases and cystic fibrosis. You will be given counselling before being inseminated with donor sperm. Patients of mine who have conceived through donor sperm have spent a long time discussing it with their partner first.

Insemination is usually done with IUI, IVF or ICSI and the success rates are the same as for those who use their partner's sperm. However, the identity of the donor will remain unknown and will only be revealed if the child, once they are aged eighteen, decides they want to trace their genetic parent. (Note: the donor, however, is not able to trace the child.)

Why IVF sometimes fails

IVF, like natural conception, does not have a 100 per cent success rate. In nature, most animals take one or two attempts to conceive. Humans are different and most couples would not expect to conceive straight away. After eleven months only 70 per cent achieve conception. Why conception is

FROZEN EMBRYOS

Your clinic may offer to freeze your embryos, use them for research or destroy them. Some couples have no problem discarding the fertilized embryos not transferred during IVF, and feel no emotional attachment. Others have difficulty knowing what to do: it can present a terrible moral dilemma. For this reason, I strongly recommend couples to think about this question in advance. On the positive side, frozen embryos are an insurance policy in case a cycle doesn't work. However, you may be expecting twins or you may have more embryos than you want children. Ultimately, you will be expected to make a decision on the remaining embryos.

relatively difficult for humans is, of course, the subject of huge debate.

With the advent of IVF we have made enormous leaps in medical science and in terms of what we can now achieve for those with fertility issues. And who knows what advances will be made in future? But it's still early days, and we have to remain realistic about our limitations.

When IVF fails, it can be yet another devastating blow for couples who have already been dealt one knock after another. Many couples ask why, and sometimes we just don't know; I have tried to put together below, however, a comprehensive list of reasons in both Chinese medicine and Western terms.

Chinese medicine

Your fertility type, as described in Chinese medicine, will affect the way in which you respond to IVF and the drugs involved in the process, which is why so much of this book relates to trying to help you correct your fertility type and reach as close as possible to the 'ideal'.

Yin Deficient types, for example, are often classified as 'poor responders' in IVF. Blood Deficient types, on the other hand, often do badly on clomid stimulation, while Heat types can suffer during IVF because of the 'heating' nature of the drugs – reducing your Heat is essential in the preparation for IVF. I encourage all my patients to consider the following questions:

- Did the follicles grow and develop evenly on each side?
- How many eggs did you produce?
- Were the embryos good quality?
- Did they grow evenly on both sides?
- How many fertilized?
- Were they able to freeze any embryos?
- How was the quality of the sperm?

- Was your partner able to produce a sample easily?
- Did they need to use ICSI?
- Did they transfer on Day 3 or 5?
- Did your endometrium thicken fully?
- Did you get an early pregnancy that failed to continue?

Chinese medicine does offer another level of understanding and often gives the patient direction and hope that they can do things for themselves, enhancing their chances for future cycles.

Sometimes, a failed cycle can demonstrate that another cycle is not a good idea, and this can be hard to take. If a patient's embryos were poor quality, for example, and there were not many produced, this can indicate a decline in Kidney Yin and does not bode well. In such cases, the patient may well do better using natural methods to improve their chances since the embryos may not withstand the rigours of IVF.

However, if there was a good number of embryos produced and/or a high level of fertilization, yet the pregnancy still failed – this may indicate that work is needed on the implantation phase. It is still worth pursuing the IVF though. If it was a case of the endometrium not thickening, looking at the information on nourishing Blood may improve it in the next cycle. But I am not in charge here, and you must work closely with your clinic to decide whether or not to keep going.

Q&A

How long should we avoid sex? At least until you have your results. The prostaglandins in sperm can make the uterus contract and this is inadvisable after transfer. There is also a risk of infection. There is quite a lot of discomfort for the woman after egg collection and it is important to let everything settle down and heal.
TIPS: if you are still sore or bloated, don't push yourself to have sex as it is important to feel comfortable in any activities that you do in the early stages. You may wish to avoid it for the first trimester or you may feel ready a whole lot sooner – go with what you feel, rather than what you think you should or shouldn't do.

Balancing your type for IVF

What I look for in a patient – as I have already said, earlier in the book – is whether there is an underlying imbalance that is causing their fertility issues and how this can be corrected. The following are the most common problems (by type) and areas you may want to work on for your next cycle of IVF.

Kidney Yin Deficiency

When the Kidney Yin is deficient (see page 259 for a description) the body generates too much heat, which then dries up the fluids and blood. This can lead to poor follicular development, high FSH levels and problems with the quality and quantity of embryos produced during an IVF cycle.

Women with this condition may also feel quite restless and agitated during an IVF cycle and suffer from night sweats. If you are Kidney Yin Deficient, it is vital to do the maximum possible preparation for IVF to ensure that the yin of the body is strong and that you can produce the best-quality embryos. I usually suggest four menstrual cycles as preparation, and you really need to see a change in both your menstrual cycle and in your FSH levels to show that the necessary rebalancing has occurred.

Kidney Yang Deficiency

You may have Kidney Yang Deficiency if your embryos appeared normal, but failed to implant. This may indicate low Yang levels as well as low progesterone levels. It is important to add warmth to your preparation and to follow the plan for Cold types and Kidney Yang Deficient types. However, you would be well advised to think about nourishing your Blood.

Blood Deficiency

A description of this type can be found on page 121. As we have already discussed, if the endometrium does not reach the requisite thickness (8mm), the embryo may fail to implant. Preparing by following the Blood Deficiency plan for four menstrual cycles is highly recommended before starting another cycle of IVF, and you should also consider working with a herbalist to improve your endometrial thickness (see page 280 for more on herbs and IVF). It is also important for you to rest and take it easy after embryo transfer to give your blood the best chance to nourish the embryo.

Damp

Damp patients (description of this type can be found on page 116) may find they bloat a lot during an IVF cycle; indeed, this group is more susceptible to OHSS (see page 304), since they already suffer with accumulation of fluids. I can often tell when Dampness presides, as the abdomen feels clammy to touch and the flesh may be lacking in tone.

There is a great deal that can be done to help if you are Damp. You need to follow the Damp-elimination plan quite strictly, and to address any low-grade infections, such as cystitis, thrush or any vaginal discharge, prior to starting a cycle of IVF will limit the problem during the cycle itself.

Qi and Blood Stagnation

Qi Stagnation types (a full description can be found on page 132) need to keep calm throughout the cycle.

Make sure your mind is on board and practise meditation and meridian tapping (see page 318) to help keep you calm. Disturbances in the flow of Qi may inhibit correct flow of Qi, and consequently blood, to the uterus. It may also make the body and cervix tense and therefore make embryo transfer difficult and painful. Relax.

For Blood Stagnation types, the issue is around preparing prior to IVF, as it is hard to affect the blood at this level during a cycle of IVF. However, you can also follow the guidelines for

Qi Stagnation throughout the IVF cycle. Acupuncture during IVF will help to keep blood moving in a gentle way.

This condition relates to antiphospholipid antibodies or 'sticky blood' (see below and Chapter 8) and may also include other blood-clotting issues.

Other factors in Western terms

- **Embryo quality** The quality of your embryos declines with age and therefore the quality of the embryos may also be affected. This is the most common reason for IVF failure in older women, but by no means the only one. The FSH is a reasonable indicator of ovarian reserve and a high FSH (over ten) may indicate that the response to IVF may be poor. In such cases, women may well be put on a high dose of stimulation drugs in an attempt to produce a higher number of embryos.
- **Endometrium problems** These are seen either in the thickness of the endometrium or in the level of scarring. Where the endometrium is too thin, some clinics will offer Viagra. Studies show a mixed outcome, however if the patient is either very Blood or Yin Deficient, putting them on Viagra does not help much. Once again, the key here is in preparation. Problems with the womb lining are quite common when three or more IUI cycles are undertaken using clomid due to the heating and drying effect it has on the body. Scarring from previous abdominal surgery or from C-sections or D&C can also interfere with implantation and the extent of the scarring will determine the embryo's ability to implant. Other problems include fibroids, polyps and a uterine septum (see Chapter Seven for more on these conditions.)
- Immune issues See Chapter Eight.
- Antiphosolipid antibodies (APA) The presence of APAs is more likely to create clotting issues and recurrent

miscarriage. They would be treated with blood thinners such as heparin and aspirin. See Chapter Eight.

- Natural killer (NK) cells These are naturally occurring cells in the uterus. Some clinics are looking at levels of NK cells in the blood and, if necessary, are treating with heparin, steroids, aspirin and sometimes IVIG (intravenous immunoglobulin). Speak to your clinic to get the most up-to-date research; see also Chapter Eight.
- Sperm quality ICSI has been the major breakthrough in treating male infertility, since it allows IVF clinics to inject sperm directly into the egg. This does improve fertilization rates in IVF, which gives the patients a larger number of embryos to choose from. However, it does not guarantee implantation.

Is the mind on board?

I have included in the section on meridian tapping, see below, some affirmations to help lower your FSH levels. In addition, there are affirmations and visualizations in Chapters Four to Seven that apply to each phase of your IVF cycle.

Yoga

The yoga sequence we use for fertility is outlined in full in Chapter One. There are additional sequences under the relevant sections of the menstrual cycle in Part Two.

Meridian tapping

Meridian tapping, also known as EFT, is a simple yet effective way of working to resolve the change on negative memories which may be contributing towards physical or emotional blocks in the here and now. It is a simple, easy-to-learn technique involving tapping meridian points on the face and upper body with your fingers, and the sequence takes just minutes.

The sequence

This sequence uses fifteen of the meridian points on the body (see diagram on page 321); it really is best to learn them off by heart, so that you know them without thinking – on 'autopilot', as it were. There is also an abridged version of eight that you can do pretty much at any time, wherever you are. You'll need to learn:

- your 'set-up statement' (this is the phrase that you repeat)
- tapping the meridian points and the sequence
- the shortcut version
- a script for your IVF treatment (you can adapt this to your own needs).

Your set-up statement

This is not an affirmation (affirmations being purely positive) because it does acknowledge that there is a negative part to the process too – that being the part we're trying to shift, of course. The statement runs as follows:

'Even though I am anxious, I deeply and completely love and accept myself.' [9]

Both negative and positive ideas co-exist here. This allows for self-acceptance – which is important when working with physical issues such as fertility. The 'set-up' also stops unconscious self-sabotage. Our inner saboteur is a voice we are all familiar with – it's the one that says, 'Eat the chocolate cake!' when we are on a diet. It is a powerful force and it can stop us from achieving our goals. The saboteur comes and goes all the time, so do the set-up each time – it will do no harm and it only takes a minute or so.

To do the set-up, take the first two fingers of one hand and tap on the side of your other hand in the place where you would deliver a karate chop. You need to apply a little pressure – about as much as when someone gives you a prod. The aim is to send a vibration of energy down that point. As you tap on this point, say your 'set-up' sentence out loud:

'Even though I _____, I deeply and completely love and accept myself.' (Fill in the blank with your issue.)

Repeat your statement three times. It may feel a bit odd the first time you try it. If you are really struggling with the 'I deeply love and accept myself' part of the sentence, try, 'I am OK' or 'I am good' or 'I am cool'. Then work towards saying, 'I deeply love and accept myself.'

Tapping the meridian points

How to tap:

- You can tap with either hand but it's probably easier to use the dominant one.
- Tap using the tips of your index and middle fingers.
- Tap solidly, but never hard enough to hurt.
- Tap around seven times on each point.

The points are as follows:

- The eyebrow – at the beginning, just above and to one side of the nose.
- The side of the eye – on the bone, bordering the outside corner of the eye.
- Under the eye – on the bone under the eye, about 2.5cm below your pupil.
- Under the nose – on the small area between the bottom of your nose and the top corner of your upper lip.
- Chin – midway between the point of your chin and the bottom of your lower lip.
- Collarbone – at the junction where the breastbone, collarbone and first rib meet. To locate it, first place your forefinger on the U-shaped notch at the top of the breastbone. From the bottom of the U, move your

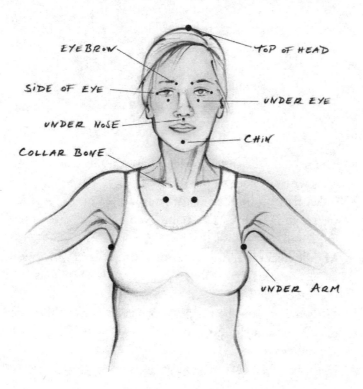

MERIDIAN TAPPING POINTS

EYEBROW

TOP OF HEAD

SIDE OF EYE

UNDER EYE

UNDER NOSE

CHIN

COLLAR BONE

UNDER ARM

finger down an inch towards your stomach, then to the left (or right) by one inch. It is at the beginning of the collarbone.

- Under the arm – on the side of the body, at a point even with the nipple (for men), or in the middle of the bra strap (for women).
- Below the nipple – for men, an inch below the nipple; for women, where the bottom of the breast meets the chest wall.
- Top of the head – on the crown of your head, spanning both hemispheres.

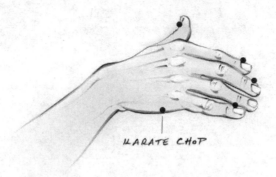

KARATE CHOP

- Thumb – on the outside edge of your thumb, at a point even with the base of the thumbnail.
- Index finger – on the side of your index finger (the side facing your thumb), at a point even with the base of the fingernail.
- Middle finger – on the side of your middle finger (the side closest to your thumb), at a point even with the base of the fingernail.
- Little finger – on the inside of your baby finger (the side closest to your thumb), at a point even with the base of the fingernail.
- Karate chop: as described above.

Note: if you tap your sequence down the body, it makes it easier to remember.

And the shortcut version is:
- beginning of the eyebrow
- side of the eye
- under the eye
- under the nose
- chin
- beginning of the collarbone
- under the arm
- top of the head.

Using tapping to support IVF

There are many ways in which tapping can be helpful during fertility treatment and IVF. In my practice, I see couples at varying stages of IVF. Often, they have a history of failed IUI or ICSI cycles. Sometimes, they may also have a history of miscarriage.

When women have a fertility history like this, they sometimes feel as if their body has failed them. This hurts their very identity as a woman. Addressing and getting rid of the negative beliefs and emotional blocks to conception, natural or otherwise, allows them to relax and rebalance, opening up the possibility of successful pregnancy in the future.

I suggest that you tap with the thoughts that are plaguing you most at this point in time:

- Even though my body has let me down...
- Even though I have failed as a mother...
- Even though all I want is to be a mother and I can't do it...
- Even though I feel useless as a woman...
- Even though this is so difficult for me, I am open to the possibility that I can sustain a happy, healthy, nine-month pregnancy easily...
- Even though I feel guilty...
- Even though I am too old...

Once you have done this, I'd like you to introduce a specific 'choice'. Why not ask your unconscious to tune into the wisdom of the generations of women before you, who conceived in order for you to be here today. It may feel strange, but trust me, there is something in it:

- 'I choose to harness the wisdom of generations before me who must have known how to conceive successfully in order for me to be here.'
- 'I look to the generations of women before me who

conceived for me to be here and I ask them to support and guide me.'

You can play around with this idea and the sentence until it feels comfortable.

There are also many ways in which, with persistence and determination, tapping can positively support the physical changes and responses that need to happen during IVF treatment. For example, if you are having an FSH test that measures your ovarian reserve, make a lower figure your 'choice'. So: 'Even though my FSH is X, I choose for it to be Y.' Start tapping once the drugs to shut the reproductive system down have been effective (the down-regulation process) and follicle stimulation begins.

I ask my patients to tap on this choice, many times during the day, as well as to use visualization techniques. Often the results are surprising. Use the choices, to help follicle stimulation and blood flow to the womb. Visualize the reproductive system as healthy and receptive to pregnancy, tapping on any blocks as and when they appear. For example:

- 'Even though I am anxious about this process, I choose to have X healthy follicles in each ovary.'
- 'Even though I can't believe this will work, I choose to produce X healthy follicles easily now.'
- 'Even though I am worried about this, I choose for my womb to be welcoming and receptive to my embryos.'
- 'Even though I am anxious about my embryos, I send them love.'

Once the embryos have been implanted in the womb, turn your attention to encouraging them to latch on, thrive, etc. Again, visualize this happening at the same time. Use your own language in the choice.

I am occasionally asked whether all of this is not just setting up false hopes. My answer is that if the outcome of the treatment is negative, a patient's disappointment is the same whether they have been positive about it or not. We are not creating a false reality, only opening the door to the possibility of success.

Meridian tapping does have a way of empowering people during treatment, so that even if it is not successful, they do at least feel they have done the best they possibly can.

Visualization
This is the guided visualization I do with my patients:

'Feel that vibration already beginning to resonate around your body, flowing through every cell, every fibre of your being, paying particular attention to those areas that need it the most right now. Enjoy that. Share this love and connection with your eggs/your sperm, so that they too can benefit from the energy of love as they prepare for fertilization easily now. Draw on the wisdom of generations of women/men before you who must have known how to conceive successfully in order for you to be here. Allow that inner wisdom to flow around every cell in your body, tuning your awareness into the future and what you can achieve. And, as your body benefits already from what it has learnt today, you can feel gratitude for the amazing being that you are and will continue to be, opening your mind to the limitless possibilities that are available to you right now.'

Qigong
This is the palm-healing exercise – for preparation and down regulation:
- Stand with your feet shoulder-width apart, shoulders relaxed, elbows out to the side and fingers directed in towards your lower abdomen, below the navel.

Concentrate on the sense of connecting with your subtle internal self. Hold this position for a while.

- Slowly raise your hands along the centre line of your body, fingers still directed inwards, as if you are tracing the movement of the subtle internal Qi. Cross your wrists as you come up and pause when you arrive at the level of the centre of your chest – your heart. Concentrate on sensing your deep heartfelt feelings.

- Slowly uncross your arms; following the Qi out from the heart, down your arms to your fingertips. With your arms outstretched at shoulder height, as if the energy reaches the horizon, pause and sense your connection with nature.

- Then slowly raise your arms above your head, as if the energy of your fingers combs through the clouds. Stand with your arms stretching upwards, as if you can touch your original source of power. Keeping your fingers pointing up to the sky, slowly lower your arms. Bring your hands down behind your head, then around your neck and point your fingertips in towards your throat. Slowly lower the hands down to the heart.

- Turn your hands to follow the contours of your ribcage, over the spleen (left-hand side of the ribcage), stomach and liver (right-hand side), moving down and round to the kidneys as you bend at the waist. Link your fingertips into the spine and follow the spine down to your tailbone, then out to the side of the hips.

- Keeping yourself relaxed at the waist, slowly lower your hands down the outside of the legs, all the way to your feet and down to the earth, sending all the heavy, tired energy down into the centre of the earth.

- Bring your hands to the inside arch of your feet, as if you are following the Qi up the inside of your calves, knees, thighs, up to your pelvis and finally returning to the starting position with your fingers pointing into your lower abdomen.

Once you have learnt this pattern of movement, simply follow without thinking and allow the Qi to lead you. When you choose to finish, always complete a full round of the exercise and close in the original position, anchoring the Qi in your lower abdomen, below the navel.

See also the infinity pattern (page 327) for the stimulation phase and the post-ovulation exercise in Chapter Seven for implantation.

Heart and Womb

Above all, I urge you to keep your connection with your Heart and what it needs. Keep the loving strong between you and your partner, be gentle with each other and take care of each other's feelings – everyone is sensitive on a journey like this, no matter how brave their face.

And try to keep the connection between the Heart and Womb strong. Imagine it: shut your eyes, place your left hand on your heart and your right hand on your womb. Feel the connection between the two; feel how the energy naturally moves between them. If you don't feel this, maybe try and imagine it as light. What colour is it? Make it a warm colour. Send the energy from your Heart deep into your Womb.

Do this as often as you need to – whenever you feel anxious, sad or ungrounded. Just connect back to your heart and remember how important it is to nourish it and your emotions. This is, after all, what makes us human.

Moving on

When IVF fails, patients are left with a difficult decision of what to do next. For some, the journey will stop here, and supporting them emotionally through this time is one of the most important parts of my job. Treating the Heart cannot be separated from the physical body, and so in many ways this is part of what we do best in Chinese medicine. See 'Childlessness,' over the page.

Other patients will decide at this point to explore other channels, specifically surrogacy and adoption.

Surrogacy

Surrogacy involves a third party who agrees to be impregnated and carry the baby for a couple who are unable to conceive themselves because of fertility issues. The surrogate may be impregnated through IVF using your embryos. Alternatively, she may carry an embryo from donor eggs and/or sperm or she may use her own eggs.

In the UK, there is still a range of legal issues surrounding surrogacy. Speak to your clinic for more information and see Resources.

Adoption

Adoption can be a complicated and drawn-out process in the UK, but is, for many, a life-enriching experience. Your local authority will want to ensure that you, the place that you live and the environment that you will bring a child up in, meet their stringent criteria.

Some couples choose to adopt from abroad, which can also be a lengthy process, as well as an expensive and frustrating one, and it is important to equip yourself with all the available facts before you head down this route. The websites at the back have details on all aspects of adopting a child.

Facing childlessness

Giving up on your dream of having a child is a painful and gradual process. It may follow a very long period of failed fertility treatments and the decision to stop trying is a heart-wrenching one. Up until this point there was always hope.

For the purposes of this book, I have spoken to a number of women about their experiences. Some told me that they really needed to *know* that the much-wanted child was not going to come. They wanted it spelled out. They had exhausted every option and they felt exhausted.

Most of them said that the moment they decided to stop brought with it a wave of emotions; some said that it even came with a tremendous amount of relief. It is, without doubt, a draining journey.

I think it's important to grieve for that child you wanted, and to allow the other emotions that go with this to come out. You may feel anger, with yourself, with the world around you, with friends who have conceived without issue. You may feel a sense of loss, not just for the child, but for the structure the whole process gave your life. You may even feel what is often described as 'a numb pain'.

Some women have described a feeling of being out of step with the rest of society and at a sudden loss as to where to direct all the energy and passion that they had been putting into fertility. Others have described feeling 'light', as if they were at an interesting time 'of new beginnings' they hadn't imagined before.

You may adapt to seeing your life in a way you never expected. I have witnessed women go on to find extraordinarily creative outlets for their passion. Some throw it into a hobby they had always thought about doing, some pack up and go round the world, some carry on as normal, but with a deeper understanding of what life is; and that in itself, can bring a new kind of optimism.

Talking it all through with a professional and with those whom you trust to listen is very important. Grieving is very much a part of healing. The pain does lessen and acceptance and peace do come. It can be a challenge to move on, but it can also seem like the natural progression.

If you feel that you are 'stuck' in one part of the grieving process or feeling one emotion particularly strongly – say, anger – I recommend that you find additional support to help you cope with your situation. (See also Resources for further reading.)

Chapter Ten

Conclusion

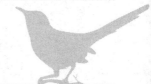

Jing, the Chinese idea of inherited health, is something you really can pass on to your children – which is why I encourage my patients to become parents from a place of health and balance.

Many couples experience something extraordinary in the course of their fertility journey. As they reassess and shift the priorities in their lives, change occurs at a deep level and, in the process, often something beautiful can emerge – an understanding of what I mean by 'a healthy conception' and everything that goes with it. I am told by many patients that engaging in the process of getting healthy for conception changed their lives for the good, making them happier, calmer individuals, with more strength, confidence and a greater appreciation of joy. As one patient said to me the other day, 'Great health is a better gift to your children than great wealth'.

Western medicine is a constantly evolving entity, absorbing from other disciplines where it sees their strengths. My colleagues, such as Tim Evans, Michael Dooley, Jeannie Yoon and Adrian Lower, are all at the very forefront of their fields in Western medicine and it is a mark of their brilliance, in my opinion, that they are so open to traditions outside their own. This doesn't mean to say, of course, that they agree with everything *I* believe – but our discussions are lively and ultimately benefit the patients we see.

What I would like to see now is further collaboration between Western medicine and outside influences. My ideal would be less IVF and more focus on pre-conception care. I would like to see younger women encouraged and educated to address their gynaecological and sexual health much earlier in their life and for this to be supported by acupuncture, good nutritional preparation and emotional support.

When we know what the problem is – be it a blocked Fallopian tube or poor sperm quality – IVF is a miracle treatment and success rates are increasing year on year. But I am uncomfortable with the use of IVF where the problem *isn't* clear. Should women really be going through highly invasive, expensive medical treatments when we have no idea why they are not conceiving? But in many cases patients (and some doctors) simply don't know that there are alternatives. And this, I believe, is where Chinese medicine (along with complementary therapies), can play a starring role. It is where there is a real opportunity to explore the benefits of 'whole-body' health, using simple and gentle treatments for the body *and* the mind.

In my clinic, this is a first-line treatment, of course, and its potency cannot be underestimated. The majority of women who come to me because they are having problems conceiving go on to conceive naturally with acupuncture and the baby-making plan I offer them, as described in this book, including adjustments to their diet, lifestyle and outlook. Some critics will say this is purely coincidental: after all, 90 per cent of couples conceive within a year of having started to try.

I am sure that in some cases it *is* a coincidence, and, if nothing else, it is great that unnecessary medical procedures were avoided by them coming to me first. But what about the cases where women who, after years of unexplained infertility, or failed IVF cycles are able to conceive following revolutionary changes to their lifestyle?

I hope that clinical trials (such as those that have shown the enormous benefits of acupuncture) will be undertaken to test our work to standards that are acceptable in Western medicine. We need to test our practices to their very limits. This will allow Chinese medicine to be integrated even further into the mainstream.

My belief in the wisdom of Chinese medicine extends beyond conception, to life in general. At the centre of its teaching is the idea of balance. That includes balancing the mind and the body and keeping them in harmony.

It is my hope that as a generation we learn to let go of rigidity in the way we think, to listen to our bodies and to our emotions. We need to appreciate our connection with the world around us: what we do to our environment, we do to ourselves. Clarity and balance in our emotional lives will have far-reaching effects. We need to strive to find peace within ourselves, and love and harmony in our relationships with others will quickly follow. We need to hold on to the basic truths about what makes us happy, content and fertile. We need to hold on to love, kindness and compassion.

Most people who have endured a struggle at some point in their lives will tell you of a new appreciation and empathy that came with it. Even the most difficult situations in life can have a positive side, and there is often opportunity within a crisis. There cannot be dark without light, day without night, joy without sorrow; it is a universal truth – the Yin and Yang of life.

I hope this book will help get the message out there.

Appendix

Yoga fertility sequence

I suggest you either record the instructions on to a tape and then play it back to yourself, or get your partner or a friend to talk you through each practice. You can practise straight from the book, but you don't want to interrupt your poses too often to look at the next instruction; you may be better off committing it to memory.

The following 'fertility' sequence and the individual poses have been devised by my colleague Uma Dinsmore-Tuli. You will find her specific recommendations for each stage of the menstrual cycle as you follow the plan in Part Three.

The maximum time to spend on this whole programme would be 110 minutes for a full, leisurely practice. However, an abbreviated version could take just fifteen minutes, or a short complete version would be about half an hour.

There is no need for any special yoga equipment other than a comfortable mat to lie on and a blanket to cover yourself in the relaxation practices. A couple of cushions are also helpful for some of the resting poses, and an eye bag.

The sequence comprises nine core practices, as follows:

- Full yogic breath and inner awareness (in super deluxe *savasana*) – five to ten minutes.
- Seed to flower: alternating between opening and protection – three to five minutes.
- *Shakti bandha:* freeing of feminine energy – three to five minutes.
- *Chandra* sequence: honouring the moon (with variations) – five to nine minutes.
- Forward bend (and restorative variations) – three to five minutes.
- Lying twist (still and moving variations) – three to five minutes.
- 'The queen' (golden womb) – five to fifteen minutes.
- *Yoga nidra* with *prana vidya* for reproductive organs – five to forty-five minutes).
- *Mudras* and meditations for honouring feminine power – three to fifteen minutes.

PRACTISING YOGA SAFELY

Don't do breathing exercises too fast, hold them for too long, or get too hot. Always aim to work at a pace that does not disrupt the natural easy flow of your breath, and at a rhythm that creates pleasant warmth, not sweaty heat.

During menstruation, avoid inversions and encourage instead the downward movement of energy. This means not to do any practice that brings the head lower than the heart, such as downward dog, and instead to do practices that provide a clear sense of being grounded and connected to the earth in order to encourage a sense of releasing the menstrual flow down and out of the body. Take your awareness into the pelvis during this time and sense which practices help you to sense an opening and release from the womb down into the vagina. Sitting practices are often effective in achieving this, or resting poses such as the Queen, but it varies from woman to woman. The focus should be on releasing energy downwards in the form of menstrual flow.

Full yogic breath and inner awareness (in super deluxe savasana) – five to ten minutes

Take time to set yourself up in simple comfort, lying on your mat with a pillow for your head, and bolster behind your knees.

1. Rest the palms of both hands flat on your belly below the navel, with thumbs touching each other. Your index fingers should also touch, to form a downward-pointing triangle, the symbol of feminine energy or *shakti*. Your fingertips should point down, and may rest on the pubic bone. This is called *yoni mudra* (the gesture of honouring the source of all) and the warmth of your hands builds a nourishing connection for your pelvic organs, directing energy towards them. If you find your elbows are off the ground it will not be relaxing to hold this *yoni mudra* without putting a cushion, block or rolled blanket beneath each elbow to support your arms.

2. With your hands in *yoni mudra*, focus on the movement of the breath and be aware of every exhalation, enabling your body to settle deeper down into the support of the earth beneath. Allow your belly to rise and fall freely with the breath, rising on inhalation and sinking on exhalation. Be especially aware of a relaxed freedom of movement in the abdomen, beneath your hands, allowing it to rise as the breath enters and sink as it leaves.

3. Allow also for the ribcage to expand sideways to accommodate a full inhalation, and then gently contract on exhalation. Watch the rhythmic pattern of movements in your belly and chest. Watch also, as your breath settles into an easy rhythm, that there are four parts to each breath. Do not force any single component of this four-part breath, but do be aware of its cyclical nature, circling back on itself with every breath you take, reminding you that the rhythm of breath is circular.

Seed to flower: alternating between opening and protection – three to five minutes

1. Lie on your back with your knees bent, feet flat on the floor under your knees. If you are comfortable without a pillow beneath your head, don't use it. Let your inner knees and ankles be touching. Have your hands on your belly in *yoni mudra*, as above.

2. As you inhale, reach both arms up, hands extending towards the ceiling and then back above your head, coming to rest on the floor above your head, at whatever width is easy for your shoulders (the wider the arms, the easier this is).

3. At the same time, as your arms move, allow your knees to drop wide out to the sides so that the soles of your feet turn towards each other and touch. Let your knees drop as wide as is comfortable. The position of the body at the fullness of the inhalation will be fully open: arms above head and knees wide.

4. As you exhale, reverse the opening movement: bring your hands back over your body to return to *yoni mudra*, and squeeze your legs closed so that your knees and ankles are touching again. By the end of the exhalation, your body thus returns to its closed position.

5. Repeat the opening movement with each inhalation, and the closing movement with each exhalation. Synchronize the movement of your body with your breath. Have your palms and fingers stretched open wide. To experience a smooth flow you will need to move your legs a lot more slowly than your arms. Time the movement so that the end of the exhalation corresponds with the fully closed position, and the moment of fullness on the inhalation corresponds with the fully open stretch.

6. When you are synchronized, pause in the open inhalation position until your breath is ready to leave. Pause in

the exhalation position until you are ready to allow
the next breath in. In this way, you become aware of
the four components of breath and allow your body to
be nourished by the breath within it, and to rest in the
fully empty, receptive place that exists when your body
is awaiting the arrival of the next breath. Do not force
either pause – just observe the natural rhythms of your
breath.

Shakti bandha: freeing of feminine energy – three to five minutes

Grinding The Mill *(chakki chalanasana)*: this is a lovely,
rhythmic pelvic circling practice that promotes flexibility and
ease of movement from the hips, while toning the nerves and
organs of the pelvis and abdomen. Its Sanskrit name means
'grinding the mill', but it works just as well to think of it as
stirring the porridge. Do not do this practice if you have high
blood pressure or acute lower-back pain.

1. Sit with your legs straight and separate them as wide as is
   comfortable. Push your heels away from you and draw
   your toes towards you. Have your spine upright and
   sit forwards on your sitting bones so that your pelvis is
   tilted to the front. Have your arms by your sides.
2. Extend your arms out in front, at shoulder height (your
   elbows can bend to allow your shoulders to slide freely
   down, away from your ears). Interlock your fingers
   so that the right thumb is on top. Imagine that you
   are holding a huge wooden spoon and that there is an
   enormous pot of porridge placed between your two heels.
3. Begin to stir the porridge clockwise, moving from your
   hips to trace large circles with your imaginary wooden
   spoon. Exhale as you move forwards into the circle,
   and inhale as you lean back out of it. One circle is one
   round. Repeat nine times, clockwise, then pause after the

ninth round and rest your arms down by your sides.

4. Raise your arms back up to shoulder height, interlock
   your fingers with the left thumb on top, and repeat the
   above steps, circling anti-clockwise. At the end of the
   ninth round, rest your arms by your sides, sit with a
   straight spine and observe your breath settling. Feel that
   the movement comes from your hips. Keep your spine
   straight throughout, but let your elbows bend. Draw
   your shoulderblades together and move them downwards
   – it should feel as if you are sliding your shoulders down
   your back. This creates a feeling of openness in your
   chest and freedom in the neck. Let your shoulders be free
   and not tense.

GRINDING THE MILL

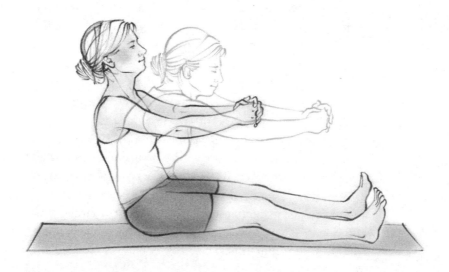

Chandra sequence: honouring the moon (with variations) – five to nine minutes

This sequence re-energizes the pelvic area and is best done in the evening. Basically, all the movements are done on the exhalation. It is a good idea to have a folded blanket or cushion under your knees throughout this practice.

1. Start from kneeling (the thunderbolt position). Bring your hands into prayer position. Press the heels of your hands together to create a straight line across your chest from elbow to elbow. Exhale.
2. Inhale as you then rise up on your knees. Exhale. Point your fingers forwards and straighten your arms out in front of you. Open your arms wide to the sides at shoulder height as you inhale.
3. Exhale as you step your left foot forwards. Allow your knee to bend at a 90-degree angle so that your left knee is directly over your left ankle. Keep your arms spread wide. Inhale. (see illustration)

HONOURING THE MOON

4. Then exhale as you bring your left arm back behind you. Look along the length of your left arm. Keep both arms straight and at shoulder height. Inhale as you return to the front. Exhale as you bring your right arm back behind you. Look along the length of your right arm. Keep both arms straight and at shoulder height. Inhale as you return to the front.
5. Exhale as you bend at the waist to lower your left arm, reaching your fingertips down towards the floor (there is no need to touch the floor, just reach towards it). Stretch your right arm up, keeping a long straight line

from your right fingertips to the left. Look up at your right hand. Inhale as you return to centre, arms wide. Exhale as you bend at the waist to bring your right arm down to reach its fingertips towards the floor. Stretch your left arm up, keeping a long, straight line from left fingertips to right. Look up at your left hand. Inhale as you return to centre, arms wide.

6. Exhale as you step your left foot back to return to the thunderbolt. Then bend at the waist to come down on to all fours for the cat pose. Have your palms flat on the floor, directly under the shoulders with fingers well spread and pointing forwards. Inhale fully as you look forwards and slightly up, lengthening through the whole spine as it arches slightly. On an exhalation, tuck your chin down right into your chest, tuck in your tailbone and suck your belly up to your spine. Your back should be rounded right over. Press the heels of your hands down into the floor and open up a space between your two shoulder blades. Inhale and look forwards again, arching your back slightly.

7. This is an adaptation of the half-moon pose: to do it from the cat pose, step your left foot off the side of your mat, and lift and straighten your knee so the side of your foot is resting on the floor. Then reach your left hand forwards and straight up above you into the air, turning your head and chest to look up at your hand, creating an open chest. Exhale and reach your arm down. Extend the arm, reaching up so that the inner part of the upper arm rests alongside your ear. Then place your hand back on the floor. Then move on to the next pose in the sequence.

Variations: I will refer back to these variations in later chapters. However, in this Moon sequence, continue from above and follow the poses through in the following order.

- **Dog pose:** Exhale, as you tuck your toes under and swing your tailbone up into the dog pose. Keep your elbows and knees strong and straight. Inhale as you raise your right leg up behind you. Exhale as you place it back on the floor. Inhale as you raise your left leg up behind you. Exhale as you place it back on the floor. Inhale.
- **Hare pose:** Exhale as you bend your knees back down to the floor in hare pose. Lower your head to the floor and extend your arms out in front of you at shoulder width. Move your knees wider to make this easier.
- **Hare–cobra pose:** Keep your hands and knees firmly rooted into the mat as you creep forwards, low along the mat, slowly bringing the front of the body into contact with the mat, and lifting your chest into the cobra pose. Return the same way you came, pushing backwards a little way up from the floor until you return to the hare pose.
- Return to the start – by rolling up through your spine, as you inhale, and raising your arms and upper body back to the vertical, keeping your ears between your arms, so that there is a continuous line from tailbone to fingertips. Keep sitting back on your heels in the thunderbolt as you exhale your hands back into the prayer position, pressing the heels of your hands together to create a straight horizontal line from elbow to elbow.
- Then repeat the sequence with the right foot forwards, starting each pair of movements with your right arm moving instead of the left. Start and finish in thunderbolt with prayer-position hands.

Forward bend (and restorative variations) – three to five minutes

Hare pose (folding forwards from kneeling to bring your forehead to the floor) is a restful forward bend if you bring your knees wide enough to make it easy and comfortable. Have a cushion or bolster in front of you for your head if you find your forehead does not easily reach the ground. Sit with a bolster between your knees if your buttocks do not readily touch your heels.

Alternatively, sit with your legs straight out, as for stirring the porridge (see page 338), and place a chair in front of you, between your legs, so that you can rest your head forwards on the seat of the chair. Put a bolster or cushion on the chair seat to make it the right height (when it is exactly perfect your lower back is completely comfortable). An alternative or additional variation is to have your legs crossed. Swap the cross of your legs halfway through the practice.

Lying twist (still and moving variations) – three to five minutes

1. Lie on the floor with your knees and feet together. Have a pillow under your head.
2. Bend your right knee, and tuck the toes of your right foot under the back of the left knee.
3. Move your left arm across your body and place the palm of your left hand on top of your right knee. Take an abdominal inhalation. On your exhalation, allow your right knee to move across the body and drop down towards the floor on the left-hand side. Once the right knee reaches the floor, let it rest there, with your hand on top. Breathe evenly in the pose and turn your head to the right if this is comfortable for your neck.
4. On an inhalation, bring your head and right knee back to the centre.

5. Repeat, with your left knee moving to the floor on the right-hand side and your head turning to the left.

6. Before settling into stillness in this pose, use a gentle rhythmic opening and closing on each side (rather like the way in which you synchronized breathing and movement in the seed to flower pose, page 337): have your arms stretched out straight on the floor in front of you at shoulder level, with the palms touching, and left arm on top.

7. As you inhale, lift your left arm up towards the ceiling and take it as far into an open stretch behind you as it will comfortably go. As you exhale, bring your arm back down again so that the palm of your left hand is resting back on top of your right hand at the end of the exhalation.

8. Repeat in time with your breath nine times, before relaxing into stillness in the twist. When you roll over to do the twist on the other side, repeat the arm movement with the other arm.

An alternative way to do this is with your hands behind your head as per the illustration.

A RESTFUL YET MOVING POSE To USE
PRE-MENSTRUALLY To HELP MOVE STAGNANT
Qi AND TONIFY THE INTERNAL ORGANS.
CALMS THE MIND.

SIDE STRETCH

'The queen' (golden womb) – five to fifteen minutes (five minutes is the minimum time for this practice).

This pose is the mother of all *asana*! It is a blissful restorative pose giving complete support and protection to the back of the body to promote an attitude of receptivity, acceptance and contentment. The sense it provides is of being completely held: and the name 'golden womb' refers to the yogic concept of the whole universe as one giant golden womb: the eternal cosmic egg within which all life is held. To be so held promotes a very regal state of comfort and ease, hence the nickname 'the queen', which is how you will feel when you are in the pose.

The pose can take a while to set up and uses lots of props but is well worth the effort, because once you are in it, you can breathe, rest or do meditative practices in total comfort for up to forty minutes.

1. First, assemble your props: a mat, cushion or folded blanket to sit on, a belt to support your sacrum, a bolster or two, plus a wall or bean bag to provide inclined support and bolsters or cushions for thighs and elbows. Additional cushions for head support can be useful, plus a blanket and eye bag.

2. Set up your back support first, putting one end of the bolster on a cushion and leaning it against a wall, using blocks, cushions or bean bags to create a comfortable angle of around 30 degrees. Sit on a cushion in front of the bolster in full butterfly, with the soles of your feet touching and your knees out to the sides. Place the belt around your lower back, just below the top rim of your pelvis, bringing the ends around to the insides of your legs; take the belt underneath your feet, so that your soles are held together without any effort. Adjust the distance between your heels and buttocks until it feels easy, then secure the belt to hold your feet in this position. Position

the belt buckle so that it does not stick into your leg.

3. Now lean back, ensuring the whole length of your spine is supported by the upright bolster: move cushions or bolsters in to support your thighs and elbows and use additional cushions or folded blankets to support your head and neck if necessary. Cover your body with a blanket if you are planning to be in the pose for more than a few minutes, and cover your eyelids with the eye bag or a scarf.

4. Rest your hands either on supports or over your belly, whichever you prefer, using *yoni mudra* (see page 337) or the heart/womb *mudra* described below. When you recline, be especially attentive to supporting your lower-back curve, and, if necessary, place an additional blanket at the bottom of the bolster. The final pose should create a feeling of complete support and comfort at all stages of pregnancy. If you are enjoying the pose, there is no reason not to remain there for up to forty minutes.

Heart/womb breath, inner silence meditation or *yoga nidra* (described below) are very beneficial to this pose. When you feel ready to come out, move slowly and gently. First, uncover yourself and draw your knees inwards, supporting the outsides of your knees with the palms of your hands.

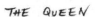

THE QUEEN

Yoga nidra with prana vidya for reproductive organs (five to forty-five minutes)

There are many different types of yogic relaxation practices. This is a shortened version of 'yogic sleep', but it is, in fact, only the body that sleeps, while the mind remains alert and attentive. It encourages the physical body to enter a deeply relaxed state, while freeing the mind from sensory input in order to access insights.

1. Before you start, the most important preliminary for an experience of *yoga nidra* is total physical comfort. Choose a lying or restorative pose, such as superdeluxe *savasana*, or the queen, and have sufficient props and covers to be warm, well supported and absolutely comfortable. Dim the lights, draw the curtains or cover your eyes. If you are uncomfortable or chilly, or if it is bright, your physical body will not relax so well or so deeply, and will provide distractions from the focus of the practice. To minimize distraction from the physical body and to deepen the quality of rest experienced in *yoga nidra*, you are usually advised to keep perfectly still throughout.

2. Once you are really comfortable, close your eyes and focus your attention on the free flow of your breath. Feel yourself settling your body into a state of stillness and quietness. Become aware of the points of contact between your body and the supports beneath.

3. Make a resolve to let your body take deep rest, while your mind remains alert and attentive. Then, prepare to carry your mental attention around your body, visiting each part of your body in turn, as if the light of your mind's attention were to come to shine briefly on each body part.

4. Now, keeping absolutely still, bring the mental attention to touch each part of your body in turn. There are very

many different systems for doing this – some are complex and some are simple. What matters is for you to choose a circuit that you can remember easily and that covers all the major body parts. Scanning down from top to bottom can work well, or you may prefer to work clockwise, or from the edges to the centre. Ensure that you include your pelvis and the organs within it on your journey around your body.

5. When you have touched each part of your body in turn with your mental attention, bring the focus of your awareness back to the rhythm of the full yogic breath. Count twenty-seven rounds of this, counting backwards down to zero. If you lose count, start again.

6. When you get to the end of the last round of breath, take your awareness into the space in front of your closed eyes and consciously there envision yourself as fully healthy, fully fertile and fully delighted with life, resting on a moonlit evening in a place you find safe and secure. Create a clear and vivid sense of yourself enjoying full health and fertility in your place of safety and security with the moon shining down upon you. Breathe consciously into this image of yourself, taking vitality and positive energy into your whole body, especially sensing the silvery light of the moon shining down upon you and soaking your whole body, right through to your reproductive organs. Let the image fade, return to the resolve you made above, and sense that your body is fully rested, and that your mind is alert and attentive.

7. To finish the practice, let your breath get a little noisier, until you can clearly hear it, waking you up. Use the sound of your breath as the bridge back to a more everyday state of awareness.

8. Stretch out through your fingers and toes, through your hands and feet. Then, stretch out through your whole

body, roll over and sit up. When you feel ready, open your eyes. Spend as much time coming out of *yoga nidra* as you did settling into it. Do not rush to sit up. Savour the effects of the practice, and move slowly and gently out of your resting position. Give yourself enough time to readjust mentally as well as physically, and make the transition from stillness to activity gradually.

9. Once you are familiar with the sequence, you may want to make your own affirmation to go with it. When you feel you have the right affirmation, use it at the start and end of the *yoga nidra* practice.

Mudras and meditations for honouring feminine power (three to fifteen minutes)

Yoni mudra (described in practice 1) is a powerful way to connect with the source of feminine energy. You can place the triangle over any part of the body that feels in need of special focus and attention. The hands usually rest very comfortably with the fingertips on the pubic bone.

1. *Hridaya mudra* (heart gesture): with hands resting palms up, lightly touch the tips of your index fingers to the tips of your thumbs. Then slide the tip of your index finger down the length of your thumb, bending it until the fingertip is tucked into the root of the thumb. Keep it in this position and touch the tip of your thumb to the tips of both your middle and ring fingers together. Your little finger remains relaxed or outstretched, whichever feels most comfortable. Traditionally, this *mudra* is held with palms up, but if it feels easier, turn them over. This hand gesture connects to the space of the heart, enhancing qualities of compassion, love and understanding.

Heart/womb *mudra*: the concept of the heart–womb connection exists both in Ayurveda, the Indian medical system closely allied with yoga, and in traditional Chinese medicine. It is an energetic link between a woman's heart and her womb. It is said to open during pregnancy, to enable a woman to nourish the child in the womb with the emotional energy of her loving heart. As an aid to building natural fertility, this practice creates a positive flow of nourishing and loving energy from heart to womb.

This special connection is the basis for a very calming and nurturing breath and awareness practice that can be done in any posture where your hands are free to rest on the front of the body. It can also be done without the hands in position, simply by bringing your mental attention to your heart and womb.

1. Sit in a comfortable and sustainable position with your eyes closed and breathe fully. Place your left palm on your chest over your heart and cover it with your right hand. Breathe freely, feeling your hands lifting and lowering with every breath. Know that every breath nourishes the love in your heart. When the heart feels fully nourished, slide your right palm down the centre line of your body until it comes to rest over your womb, resting your hand on your belly, at whatever height seems to provide a strong connection with your womb.

2. Exhaling, settle the focus of your attention into your womb, feeling warmth where your right palm rests on your belly. Inhaling, move your mental awareness from your belly up to your heart, feeling warmth where your left palm rests on your chest.

3. Exhaling, send your mental awareness back down from your heart to your womb. Continue with an easy rhythm of breath, moving your awareness from your womb (right palm) to your heart (left palm) with each inhalation, and sending awareness from heart to womb with each exhalation.

4. Sit breathing with this awareness for as long as you feel comfortable (maybe, with practice, up to twenty minutes). When you are ready, slide your right hand back up along the centre line of your body until it covers your left hand, and bring your palms together at your chest.

5. Conclude the practice with the affirmation: 'With great respect and love, I honour my heart, my inner teacher.' Repeat three times, either aloud or in your head. Breathe three more rounds, then open your eyes.

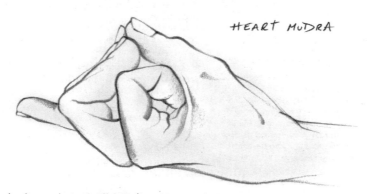

HEART MUDRA

A GOOD HAND GESTURE TO USE WHEN FEELING
OVERWHELMED WITH WORRIES. GOOD FOR SETTLING
THE HEART ENERGY AND USING WITH YOUR MEDITATIONS.

References

Introduction

[1] http://www.yuantmc.co.uk/clinic/john.htm.

[2] Emma's technique is developed from Emotional Freedom Technique, a new therapy developed in America using the ancient acupuncture points of Chinese medicine.

[3] http://www.asante-academy.com/mcintyre.htm.

Chapter One

[1] Dr Gowri Motha and Karen Swan, *Gentle Birth Method*, Thorsons, 2004.

[2] The journal *Regulatory, Interface and Comparative Physiology* published a study entitled 'Effects of acute and chronic sleep on immune modulation of rats' in 2007. Rats were deprived of sleep for 24 hours and showed a 20 per cent decrease in white blood cell count compared with the control group, which is a significant change in the immune system.

[3] 'Effects of Sleep Deprivation, nicotine and selenium on wound healing in rats', *International Journal of Neuroscience*, 2004.

[4] Professor Frank Gilliland, professor of preventative medicine, Keck School of Medicine, University of Southern California.

[5] Ibid.

[6] Marcus Pembrey, an epigenetics specialist and director of genetics at the Avon Longitudinal Study of Parents and Children in Bristol, UK, quoted in the *New Scientist*, April 2005.

[7] Dr Neil Stanley quoted by BBC News in the 'Scrubbing Up' health column, 11 February 2009.

[8] Banks S, et al., 'Behavioral and physiological consequences of sleep restriction', *Journal of Clinical Sleep Medicine*, 3:519, 2007.

[9] For more information, see Pat Thomas, *Skin Deep: The Essential Guide to What's in the Toiletries and Cosmetics You Use*, 2008 and Pat Thomas, *Healthy Happy Baby: The Essential Guide to a Toxin-free Baby*, 2008 both published by Rodale/Pan Macmillan.

[10] The study looked at a group of men in Aberdeen, Scotland and was published in *Andrology*, 2007. It is referenced in Peter Deadman, 'The Treatment of Male Subfertility with Acupuncture', *Journal of Chinese Medicine*, No. 88, October 2008.

[11] Anogenital distance is the distance between the anus and the base of the penis. If this distance is shorter than average it is taken to be a sign of 'male feminization'.

[12] Cryptorchidism is the absence of one or both testes from the scrotum.

[13] Peter Deadman, op. cit.

[14] Dr Jean Ginsburg, Royal Free Hospital, London, the *Lancet*, 22 January 1994.

[15] Dr Andrew Olshan, University of North Carolina, Chapel Hill *US News & World Report*, 14 December 1992.

[16] Robert J Norman et al. The *Lancet Vol 370*, issue 9588, pp. 685-697, 25th August 2007

[17] Robert J. Norman et al., 'Improving reproductive performance in overweight/obese women with effective weight management, *Human Reproduction Update*, vol. 10, No. 3, pp. 267–80, 2004.

[18] Ibid.

[19] Ibid.

[20] Daverick Leggett, *Recipes for Self-Healing*, Meridian Press, 1999.

[21] Ibid.

22 Overall the most common cause of maternal death.

23 According to a report published by the Confidential Enquiries into Maternal Deaths (CEMACH) in 1997, more than half of the 295 women who died during or after pregnancy between 2003 and 2005 were overweight or obese.

24 University of Texas researchers interviewed over 15,000 new mothers over 15 years and found a link between obesity at the time of conception and birth defects. Their findings are published in the *Journal Archives of Pediatrics and Adolescent Medicine.*

25 According to an American report published in 2007 by the *Journal Obstetrics & Gynecology.*

26 Researchers at the Division of Research, Kaiser Permanente, Northern California found an increased incidence of miscarriage in women who drank caffeine in the form of coffee, tea, fizzy drinks, hot chocolate or caffeinated soda compared to women who drank no caffeine. Dr De-Kun Li et al., 'Maternal caffeine consumption during pregnancy and the risk of miscarriage', *American Journal of Obstetrics and Gynecology*, 199(5):e 13–14, November 2008.

27 Daverick Leggett, op. cit.

28 Ibid.

29 Cited by Peter Deadman, 'How to be Healthy: Traditional Chinese Teachings and Modern Research', *Journal of Chinese Medicine*, No. 78, June 2005.

30 Kate Cook, The Nutrition Coach *www.thenutritioncoach.co.uk.*

31 Evening primrose should not be taken if you have had hormonal-dependent breast cancer.

32 *Statistics on Alcohol:* England, 2009. The document is available from The Information Centre, a division of the NHS *www.ic.nhs.uk/pubs/alcohol09.*

33 Drs William J. Pizzi, June E. Barnhart, et al., Department of Psychology, Northeastern Illinois University, Chicago, Illinois, *Neurobehavioral Toxicology* vol. 2:1–4, 1979.

34 Dr Madelon Price, 'Aspartame Causes Infertility – Reply', Mission Possible files, *www.dorway.com/possible.html*, 1997.

35 M. Miller et al. 'Impact of cinematic viewing on endothelial function', *Heart*, 92: 261–2, Feb 2006.

36 Cited by Peter Deadman, 'How to be Healthy: Traditional Chinese Teachings and Modern Research', *Journal of Chinese Medicine*, No. 78, June 2005.

37 Ibid.

38 Ibid.

39 Andrew L. Geers et al. 'Effects of Affective Expectations on Affective Experience: The Moderating Role of Optimism-Pessimism', *Personality and Social Psychology Bulletin*, Vol. 28, No. 8, 1026–39, 2002.

40 David R. Hamilton, *How Your Mind Can Heal Your Body*, Hay House, 2008.

41 Ed Diener uses this survey in his article 'Wealth Does Not Create Individual Happiness and it Doesn't Build a Strong Country, Either', *Psychological Science in the Public Interest*, September 2004.

42 David R. Hamilton, op. cit.

43 James M. Kilner et al., 'Functional connectivity during real vs. imagined visuomotor tasks: an EEG study', *NeuroReport*, Vol. 15, No. 4, 637–42, March 2004.

44 Both Sue Beer and Emma Roberts have thoroughly studied all Gary Craig's educational materials and have personally trained and presented with him. Whilst they feel enormous gratitude and respect for Gary, their views and the author's do not necessarily reflect those of Gary Craig or EFT. However, we highly recommend the thorough study of the complete and standardized trainings offered at *www.emofree.com.*

45 In November 2008, the journal *Behavioural Brain Research* published the results of a joint MIT-Harvard Medical School clinical study testing the effects of acupuncture as a tool for pain relief. The study used functional magnetic resonance imaging (fMRI) and positron emission tomography (PET) to examine the effects of acupuncture in relieving pain on the brain. The study concluded that, 'the reduction in pre- and post-treatment pain ratings was significantly greater in the acupuncture group when compared to the placebo group' (Dougherty et al., p.3).

46 A Swedish study of 21 women with menopausal hot flushes found that acupuncture significantly reduced symptoms. Cited in Zaborowska E. et al., 'Effects of acupuncture, applied relaxation, estrogens and placebo on hot flushes in postmenopausal women: an analysis of two prospective, parallel randomised studies.' *Climacteric*, 10(1):38–45, 2007.

47 The Cochrane Library published in 2009 a review of 40 separate international studies comparing the effects of acupuncture against a placebo and traditional anti-sickness drugs in treating nausea and vomiting after surgery. Those who had received acupuncture or stimulation of the point P-6 had the

same level of reduction in nausea and vomiting as those using anti-emetic (anti-sickness) drugs.

[48] In 2008, the British Medical Journal online published results they had collated from seven trials carried out in Western countries with a total of 1,366 women. The collated results showed that acupuncture during IVF increased by 65 per cent the chance of becoming pregnant; an 87 per cent increase in continuing pregnancy and a 91 per cent increase in live births.

[49] The British Acupuncture Council is at *www.acupuncture.org.uk*. You can also get advice on medical practitioners who use acupuncture from the British Medical Acupuncture Society *www.medical-acupuncture.co.uk*.

[50] Many women use a point just above the ankle to intensify contractions during labour, for example.

[51] Jane Lyttleton, *Treatment of Infertility With Chinese Medicine*, Churchill Livingstone, 2004, p. xv.

Chapter Two

[1] Giovanni Maciocia *The Foundations of Chinese Medicine: A Comprehensive Text for Acupuncturists and Herbalists*, Churchill Livingstone.

Chapter Three

[1] An Australian acupuncturist friend complains bitterly about the British weather: 'I arrive at Heathrow and the cellulite arrives on my thighs!' Cellulite favours damp climates making it hard to shift. Damp slows down the way we break down and assimilate our food, overloading our digestive system.

[2] Jane Lyttleton says: 'Interestingly people with Damp constitutions make poor use of the fluid they imbibe. Unlike Yin-deficient types who can't hold liquid in their tissues. Damp people hold too much fluid in their tissues, which become boggy and congested. The lack of easy fluid movement in and out of the cells means that as a vehicle for nutritional factors and wastes it is most inefficient.'

[3] Daverick Leggett, *Recipes For Self-Healing*, Meridian Press.

Chapter Four

[1] R. Pipitone, G. Gallup Jr, 'Women's voice attractiveness varies across the menstrual cycle', *Evolution and Human Behavior*, Vol. 29, Issue 4, pp. 268–74.

[2] An increasing amount of research is being done on women's attitudes towards their menses. Researchers found that young women were choosing 'menstrual suppression' in the form of oral contraceptives because among other things they felt ashamed of their periods. Articles on the subject include: 'To bleed or not to bleed: young Women's attitudes towards menstrual suppression', *Women Health* 2003; 'The need to bleed: women's attitudes and beliefs about menstrual suppression', *Journal of the American Academy of Nurse Practitioners*. 2004; 'Young Women's attitudes towards the continued use of oral contraceptives', *Health Care for Women International*, 2008.

Chapter Five

[1] Jane Lyttleton, *Treatment of Infertility with Chinese Medicine*, Churchill Livingstone, 2004.

Chapter Six

[1] Toni Weschler, *Taking Charge of Your Fertility*, Vermilion, 1995, p. 371.

Chapter Seven

[1] I discuss Yin Deficiency, which is an advanced state, in more detail in Chapter Nine.

[2] This also applies to Yang Deficiency.

[3] She even wrote a leaflet for the Royal Society For The Prevention of Accidents in Great Britain, in which she advised affected women to 'understand, recognize and sensibility adjust their lives', by not driving a car for any great distance around the time of menstruation.

[4] Anna Reynolds, who killed her mother while suffering from PMS and postnatal depression, was freed on appeal after Dalton provided evidence. She also testified for Nicola Owen, an arsonist, whose crimes coincided with a certain point in her monthly cycle, and saw her acquitted. On another occasion she had the sentence of a woman who ran over her boyfriend reduced to manslaughter, on the grounds that she had 'diminished responsibility'. Again the woman suffered from severe PMS. She had not eaten for eight hours before committing the crime and her period arrived the day after.

[5] Marilyn Glenville, *Natural Solutions to Infertility: How to increase your chances of conceiving and preventing miscarriage*, Piatkus, 2000. Reproduced with permission.

[6]   Bernard C. Gines, 'Cultural Hypnosis of the Menstrual Cycle', *New Concepts of Hypnosis*, George Allen Press, 1953.

Chapter Eight

[1]   These statistics were up to date at the time of going to press (2009) and available at *www.hfea.gov.uk*.

[2]   Michael Dooley, *Fit For Fertility: Overcoming Infertility And Preparing For Pregnancy*, Hodder Mobius, 2006.

[3]   Professor Lesley Regan is a good source on recurrent miscarriage. See *Miscarriage: What Every Woman Needs To Know*, Orion, 2001.

[4]   Jane Lyttleton, *Treatment of Infertility with Chinese Medicine*, Churchill Livingstone, 2004.

[5]   Clifford K., Raj R., Regan., 'Future pregnancy outcome in unexplained recurrent first trimester miscarriage' *Human Reproduction* Vol.12 (2) 387–9, 1997.

[6]   Liddell H., Pattison N., Zanderigo A. 'Recurrent miscarriage – outcome after supportive care in early pregnancy', *The Australian and New Zealand Journal of Obstetrics & Gynaecology*: 31:4: 3210, 1991.

[7]   Chungui fanlu Siku quanshu (Chapter 8) quoted by Heiner Fruchauf, 'All Disease Comes From the Heart: The Pivotal Role of the Emotions in Classical Chinese Medicine', *The Journal of Chinese Medicine*, No. 90, June 2009, p. 26.

Chapter Nine

[1]   Eric Manheimer, GrantZhang, Laurence Udoff, Aviad Haramati, Patricia Langenberg, Brian M Berman, Lex M. Bouter, 'Effects of acupuncture on rates of pregnancy and live birth among women undergoing in vitro fertilisation: systematic review and meta- analysis', *British Medical Journal*, 15 Feb 2008. See also Wolfgang Paulus, 'Influence of Acupuncture on the pregnancy rate in patients who undergo assisted reproductive therapy', *Fertility and Sterility*, Vol. 77, April 2002.

[2]   The HFEA is the UK's independent regulator overseeing the use of gametes and embryos in fertility treatment and research. *www.hfea.gov.uk*.

[3]   According to figures published by the HFEA *www.hfea.gov.uk*.

[4]   *BMJ*, op cit.

[5]   Dr Fedon Alexander Lindberg, in his book *The Greek Doctor's Diet*, Rodale, 2005, pp. 21–3.

[6]   Research from the University of Michigan found that city life itself impairs our ability to think. A short time in a crowded street can, according to the study, weaken memory function and reduce self-control. In contrast, nature has a positive impact on the brain: hospital patients who can see trees recover quicker; women living in council houses are more focused if they have a view of a grassy courtyard. See: Marc Berman et al. 'The Cognitive Benefits of Interacting with Nature', *Psychological Science* 2008, vol. 19, No. 12.

[7]   According to a report for the HFEA in 2005, updated in 2008.

[8]   The HFEA has restricted the number of embryos that can be transferred in IVF to a maximum of two for women under 40; and three for women aged 40 or over who are using their own eggs (for those using donated eggs, the maximum is two because these eggs will be from donors who are not older than 35).

[9]   You can add the problem you wish to confront, e.g. 'Even though I am having trouble conceiving.'

Resources

Contributors to the book

My panel of experts comprised the following, to whom I am extremely grateful:

Mr Michael Dooley Consultant obstetrician and gynaecologist and author. Founder of The Poundbury Clinic

Dr Tim Evans Private GP and GP to the Royal Household

Mr Adrian Lower Consultant gynaecologist and fertility expert based in Central London

Jane Lyttleton Chinese medicine practitioner and author based in Australia *www.acupunctureivf.com.au*

Jani White Acupuncturist specializing in fertility and pregnancy and diet dynamics. For all things concerned with having children. *www.naturechild.co.uk*

Miss Jeannie Yoon Consultant obstetrician and gynaecologist based in Central London

Emma Roberts – pioneer of EFT and Meridian Tapping in the UK; she runs the EFT Centre with Sue Beer. *www. theeftcentre.com*

Kate Cook BA Hons, Dip ION, MBANT – nutritional therapist, director of The Nutrition Coach and author of several books on nutrition. *www.thenutritioncoach.co.uk* *kate@thenutritioncoach.co.uk*

Uma Dinsmore-Tuli – yoga teacher and author based in London who specializes in fertility, pregnancy and post-natal yoga. *www.sitaram.org*

John Tindall – expert in the practice of qigong in various forms and an acupuncturist and expert in Chinese Medicine.
The Yuan Clinic *www.yuantmc.co.uk*

Daverick Leggett – Shiatsu practioner, qigong teacher and author of several Chinese dietry books. All Daverick's work is available from *www.meridianpress.net*

Useful contacts

Emma Cannon *www.emmacannon.co.uk*

A Healthy Conception
My London clinic and website
www.ahealthyconception.co.uk
Telephone: 07531 916 121

The Birth Company
This is a leading women's pregnancy
care, childbirth and gynaecology clinic
based in Harley Street, London. Emma
Cannon runs a satellite clinic from The
Birth Company.
www.thebirthcompany.co.uk

AceBabes
For support on pregnancy following
fertility treatment, multiple births
and donor conception for donors and
recipients. *www.acebabes.co.uk*
Telephone: 0845 838 1593

**British Infertility Counselling
Association (BICA)**
BICA aims to promote high-quality,
accessible counselling services for those
with fertility problems. *www.bica.net*
Telephone: 01744 750 660

Infertility Network UK (INUK)
Charity providing practical and
emotional support for people
experiencing difficulties in conceiving.
www.infertilitynetworkuk.com
Telephone: 08701 188 088

**HFEA (Human Fertilization &
Embryology Authority)**
The HFEA is the UK's independent
regulator, overseeing the use of gametes
and embryos in fertility treatment and
research. *www.hfea.gov.uk*

**NICE (National Institute for Clinical
Excellence)**
An independent organization responsible
for providing national guidance on
promoting good health and preventing
and treating ill health. *www.nice.org.uk*

British Acupuncture Council
This is the UK's main regulatory
body for the practice of traditional
acupuncture by over 2400
acupuncturists. *www.acupuncture.org.uk*
Telephone: 020 8735 0400

**Acupuncture Research Resource Centre
(ARRC)**
ARRC is a specialist resource for
acupuncture research information
funded by the *British Acupuncture
Council (BAcC)* and hosted by *Thames
Valley University's Centre for
Complementary Healthcare and
Integrated Medicine (CCHIM)*. It
was established in 1994 by the British
Acupuncture Council in partnership with
the *Foundation for Traditional Chinese
Medicine (TCM)*, a research charity.
www.acupunctureresearch.org.uk
Telephone: 020 8209 4277

Oxford Medical Supplies
Sells moxibustion and acupuncture
supplies.
www.oxfordmedicalsupplies.co.uk

AcuMedic
A Chinese medicine suppliers where you
can buy books, charts and moxibustion
supplies.
Telephone: 020 7388 5783

Neals Yard Remedies
For information on essential oils and
some herbs.
www.nealsyardremedies.com

British Osteopathic Association
Telephone: 01582 488455
www.osteopathy.org

The Register of Chinese Herbal Medicine
The Register of Chinese Herbal Medicine is a register set up to regulate the practice of Chinese Herbal Medicine (CHM) in the UK. *www.rchm.co.uk*

Acupuncture Childbirth Team (ACT) and Acupuncture Fertility Network (AFN). For more information about ACT & AFN please log on to
www.actlondon.co.uk

Yoga web resources

Sitaram Yoga *www.sitaram.org*

Yoga Biomedical Trust at the Yoga Therapy Centre (London):
www.yogatherapy.org

Yoga Therapy Centre (international trainings): *www.yogatherpycenter.org*

British Wheel of Yoga
www.bwy.org.uk

Satyananda Yoga Centre (and Satyananda teachers worldwide)
www.syclondon.com

Birthlight *www.birthlight.com*

Other web resources

For help with charting, visit *http://www.fertilityplus.org/faq/bbt/bbt.html* and *www.fertilityfriend.com* both these websites help you chart your menstrual cycle and pin point your most fertile time

http://www.surrogacyuk.org For more information on surrogacy.

www.direct.gov.uk/en/Parents Adoptionfosteringandchildrenincare/ index.htm For advice and information on adoption and fostering.
www.adoptionuk.org
www.adoptchild.co.uk

Suggested integrated practitioners working in infertility

Michael Dooley FRCOG
Consultant Gynaecologist
Tel: 0870 240 8745
www.mdooley.co.uk

Mr Adrian Lower FRCOG
Consultant Gynaecologist
The Women's Health Partnership Ltd
30 Devonshire Street,
London W1G 6PU
Tel: 020 7486 2440
Fax: 020 7487 4488
aml@adrianlower.com

Jeannie Yoon
Consultant Obstetrician and Gynaecologist
132 Harley Street
London W1G YJX,
and The Lister Hospital
Chelsea Bridge Road
London SW1W 8RH
Tel: 020 7730 2383

Nanette Greenblatt
Artist and life coach
Intuitive Consulting
art@makingart.co.uk

Suggested reading

Rachel Black and Louise Scull, *Beyond Childlessness*, Rodale, 2006.

Uma Dinsmore-Tuli, *Mother's Breath*, Hodder, 2006.

Uma Dinsmore-Tuli, *Teach Yourself Yoga for Pregnancy and Birth*, Hodder, 2007.

Michael Dooley FRCOG, *Fit for Fertility*, Hodder Mobius, 2006.

Bob Flaws and Honora Wolfe, *Prince Wen Hui's Cook: Chinese Dietary Therapy*, Paradigm, 1983.

Paul Gilbert, *The Compassionate Mind*, Constable, 2009.

Marilyn Glenville, *Natural Solutions to Infertility*, Piatkus, 2000.

Dr Jerome Groopman, *The Anatomy of Hope*, Simon & Schuster, 2004.

David R. Hamilton RhD, *How Your Mind Can Heal Your Body*, Hay House, 2008.

Angela Hicks, *The Five Laws for Healthy Living*, Thorsons, 1998.

Daverick Leggett, *A Guide to the Energetics of Food, Based on the Traditions of Chinese Medicine* (wall chart), Meridian Press, 1995.

Daverick Leggett, *Helping Ourselves: Guide to Traditional Chinese Food Energetics*, Meridian Press, 1994.

Daverick Leggett, *Recipes for Self-Healing*, Meridian Press, 1999.

Dr Fedon Alexander Lindberg, *The Greek Doctor's Diet*, Rodale, 2005.

Jane Lyttleton, *Treatment of Infertility with Chinese Medicine*, Churchill Livingstone, 2004.

Giovanni Maciocia, *Obstetrics and Gynaecology in Chinese Medicine*, Churchill Livingstone, 1997.

Giovanni Maciocia *The Foundations of Chinese Medicine: A Comprehensive Text for Acupuncturists and Herbalists*, Churchill Livingstone, 1997.

Christiane Northrup MD, *Women's Bodies Women's Wisdom*, Bantam, 2006.

Paul Pitchford, *Healing with Wholefoods*, North Atlantic Books, 1993.

Anne E. Walker, *The Menstrual Cycle*, Routledge, 1997.

Toni Weschler, MPH, *Taking Charge of Your Fertility*, Vermilion, 2003.

Merryl Winstein, *Your Fertility Signals*, Smooth Stone Press, 2003.

The Journal of Chinese Medicine (www. jcm.co.uk). Lots of Chinese medicine content including free articles and a free research database, plus a vast Chinese medicine and acupuncture book and products shop.

Books on the Hay Diet
Josephine Boyer and Katherine Cowdin,
*Hay Dieting: Menus and Recipes for
All Occasions* (with a foreword by Dr
William Howard Hay), Scribner, 1934.

Jackie Habgood, *The Hay Diet Made
Easy: A Practical Guide to Food
Combining With Advice on Medically
Unrecognised Illness*, Souvenir Press,
1997.

William Howard Hay, *Health Via Food*.
Ed. and rev. by Rasmus Alsaker, with a
special introduction by Oliver Cabana,
Jr. First printing, June, 1929; Tenth
printing, February, 1933. East Aurora,
New York, Sun-Diet Health Foundation.

William Howard Hay, *Weight Control*.
New York: Hay System, 1935.

Kathryn Marsden, *The Food Combining
Diet: Lose Weight and Stay Healthy
with the Hay System*, Thorsons, 1993.

Alexandra Pope, *The Wild Genie: The
Healing Power of Menstruation*, Sally
Milner, 2001.

Index

C

caffeine 58, 129, 169, 182, 210

cervical mucus 15, 94–5, 118, 138, 150, 178, 180, 181, 202, 206, 285

chemicals 43–5, 46, 48, 66, 197, 265

chi *see* Qi

chicken soup 48, 50–1, 103, 114, 125, 134, 159, 167, 171, 301

Chinese medicine 11–13, 16–17, 18, 26, 57, 81–2, 88, 225, 227, 310–11 *see also* acupuncture; Blood Deficient; Blood Stagnant; Cold; Damp; diet; fertility; Heart and Womb; Heat; menstrual cycle; Qi and Qi Stagnant; Yang and Yang Deficient; Yin and Yin Deficient

chlamydia 250

Clomid 139, 140, 257, 283, 284–5, 286–7, 313, 317

coffee 58, 105, 126, 139, 167, 293

Cognitive Behavioural Therapy 68–9

Cold 65, 92, 93, 95, 126, 155, 196, 227
diet 113, 114, 115, 116, 140, 159, 160, 185, 188, 208, 227
exercise 114, 115, 116, 188
menstrual cycle 113, 146, 159, 208, 218, 227
symptoms 99, 100, 101, 103, 104, 112–13, 115, 116 *see also* warming

conception *see* fertility

contraceptive pill 95, 119, 130, 162, 221

D

dairy products 49, 59, 119, 120, 162, 164, 208

Dalton, Dr Katharina 219, 220, 221

Damp 56, 59, 65, 95, 162, 188, 197, 209, 218, 298, 316
acupuncture 119, 206, 209
associated illnesses 117, 118, 119, 155, 162, 304, 316
and Cold 104, 117, 162, 228

diet 118, 119, 120–1, 140, 162–5, 170, 185, 208–9, 227–8
and Heat 100, 102, 117, 120, 127, 155, 162, 228
menstrual cycle 118, 162, 208–9, 218, 227–8
PCOS 116, 117, 118, 259, 285
symptoms 97, 99, 100, 101, 102, 103, 117, 118, 209

Deadman, Peter 46, 68, 69

diet 12, 31, 39, 47–54, 57, 60, 61, 63–5, 102, 146, 158, 172, 181, 224, 239, 265, 274, 293
and Blood Deficient 121, 122, 124, 125, 140, 167–8, 189, 210
and Blood Stagnant 137, 140, 171, 230–1
and Cold 113, 114, 115, 116, 140, 159, 160, 161, 185, 188, 208, 227
and Damp 118, 119, 120–1, 140, 162–5, 185, 188, 197, 208–9, 227–8
eating disorders 53–6
fats 49–50, 52–3, 59
fatty acids 52, 62, 65, 168, 203, 221, 223, 296
fish 62, 65, 169, 185, 223, 230, 296
and Heat 128, 129, 140, 169–70, 189, 211, 229
IVF 59, 295–6, 298, 299, 301, 302
menstrual cycle 182, 184–5, 186–88, 203, 220, 221, 223
Qi and Qi Stagnant 132, 134–35, 170, 204, 230
raw food 49, 65, 113, 116, 159, 163, 169, 226
Yang and Yang Deficient 132, 204
Yin and Yin Deficient 139, 149
see also alcohol; digestion; recipes; water

digestion 47, 48, 49, 59, 60, 99, 100, 101, 112, 117, 118, 119, 125, 129, 296

Dinsmore-Tuli, Uma 42, 83, 174

Dooley, Michael 17, 18

drugs, recreational 66, 129, 197, 201

dysmenorrhoea 155

Acknowledgements

To my family: Roger, Lily and Violet. Thank you for indulging me and giving me the space to do this – I am blessed.

To Charlotte Edwardes, for so beautifully bringing alive the ideas that have been in my head for so long; and Liz Gough, for seeing the potential – it's been thrilling. And to Brigid Moss and Anne Newman for their help in the conception and editing process, respectively. Thanks also to Emma Ashby for the layout and Juliet Percival for the illustrations.

Emma Roberts, Uma Dinsmore-Tuli, John Tindall – thank you for your heartfelt contributions which I am honoured to put in my book. Thank you Jeannie Yoon, Adrian Lower, Michael Dooley and Tim Evans and all the other medical professionals who support this approach.

To Kerry Marshall, my loyal and calming partner and friend, Michael McIntyre (herbalist), Jacqueline Schirmer (osteopath/Pilates), Kate Cook (nutritional therapist) and Kate Freemantle (acupuncturist).

My thanks to Jani White, Isobel Dunnet, Camilla Festing, Victoria Wells and Daniella Margulies for their nourishing contributions, and to Jane Lyttleton, Peter Deadman and Daverick Leggett for their inspiring and influential work. And Peta Martin, for helping me see what I needed to at the time I needed to see it.

The pages of this book are imbued with the spirit of all of you.

And lastly, to my patients: thank you for trusting me to work so intimately with you and to share your incredible journey towards parenthood. I am always humbled when asked to help. In the words of Oliver Sacks: 'Every day my patients lead me to questions and every day my questions lead me to patients.'